lympho mania

A Mostly True Account
of Life, Love, and Lymphoma

Gregg Goldman

ISBN: 978-1-963569-44-5 (hard cover)
        978-1-963569-45-2 (soft cover)

Edited by: Melissa Long

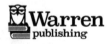

Published by Warren Publishing
Charlotte, NC
www.warrenpublishing.net
Printed in the United States

For Cali

Look for the silver lining
Whene'er a cloud appears in the blue
Remember, somewhere the sun is shining
And so the right thing to do
Is make it shine for you

A heart full of joy and gladness
Will always banish sadness and strife
So always look for the silver lining
And try to find the sunny side of life

—"Look for the Silver Lining," music
by Jerome Kern, lyrics by B. G. DeSylva

Yes, we're in deep doodoo,
Deep, deep doodoo.
So ask yourself what can you do
When the doodoo
Gets so deep?

—"Deep Doodoo," music and lyrics by Tom Lehrer

INTRODUCTION

Everyone told me journaling helps. They all swore by it, those yoga-loving, kale-eating meditators. So, when everything hit the fan, and I needed something therapeutic, I gave it a shot.

I hated it.

I'm a lefty with terrible handwriting. Ten minutes in, the side of my hand was covered with ink, and I was cramping up. I started typing to get my thoughts down quicker, but something was still missing. I don't know what possessed me to do so, but as soon as I changed to more of a storytelling perspective and less of a "Dear Diary" style, it clicked. I began typing like a madman, and writing became therapeutic.

Ironically, toward the end of this whole mess, I was reading Stephen King's book, *Billy Summers*. I haven't missed a book by Mr. King since I discovered *Christine* and *Pet Sematary* back in the eighties. I've read what I consider his *magnum opus, The Stand,* no less than five times. I just keep coming back to it, like a comfy jacket.

Anyway, the main character in *Billy Summers* begins writing for the first time too. Being an author is Billy's cover story while on a job, but he really gets into writing about his past. Billy becomes enamored with the process and starts thinking about writing when he's not writing. When he is writing, he's in the zone, cranking out page after page and vividly reliving his past. It is all very therapeutic for Billy as he sorts through some difficult memories.

As I read the book, I was astounded by the coincidence and the accuracy. Since this was just as I was completing my project, I could identify so closely with Billy's experience. I'd also never read anything about the writing process until then, and it was just uncanny, but not surprising, how Mr. King had nailed it. At some point in Billy's writing, he comes to an anecdote involving the M151 optical rifle scope. He must decide whether or not to describe it in his writing. You see, Billy knows all about the M151 scope, so if he is truly writing a journal for himself, he merely needs to mention it. But if he does describe the scope, its history, its benefits, then he is acknowledging he is also writing for someone else. Some *other reader.* It is a crossroad.

That happened early on in my "journaling." Like Billy, I moved forward in a descriptive manner. I still told myself it was just for me. Between us, I secretly hoped it wasn't.

And now, all these months later, our story—the story of my wife Cali's journey through hell as I held on for dear life—has been written. Well, a lot has happened since, but this is the story of that moment in time. I won't lie: There is a lot wrong in this book. There's a part about a robotic needle biopsy that is, as Cali has now pointed out several times, incorrect. Her hysterectomy was partially done by a robot, not the needle biopsy. But I'm leaving that in, along with a million other errors about when things happened, medical facts, people's personal history, and quite possibly my own kids' names, because (a) who gives a shit, and (b) this entire story is filtered through my fuzzy brain with its barely firing synapses, and that's all part of the ride.

My wish is for our story to help just one person cope with their feelings and experiences as a caregiver. I suppose there are many stories we don't hear. Tragedies that are too great for the survivors to retell. The exact same week Cali was diagnosed, our friend's father was as well. He just passed away yesterday. In that same amount of time, his story ended very differently. I cannot even imagine what that must have been like for his family and friends. Quite frankly, you wouldn't be reading this if things had gone differently for us. At the very least, there certainly wouldn't be the same amount of levity. I'm sure I would have quit writing halfway through if things had taken a turn for the worse.

Sadly, yet thankfully, I am very much aware things could have gone differently. But this is our story. I hope you enjoy it.

Gregg Goldman
September 27, 2021

CHAPTER 1

Bad News in Westchester County

Ijumped when my cell phone rang, even though I was expecting the call. I usually kept my phone on silent but didn't want to accidentally miss the vibration, so I had turned on the ringer. And still, it surprised me.

I was sitting in the CVS parking lot across the street from the hospital, where I had dropped off my wife, Cali. It was February 24, 2021, and due to COVID-19, visitors were not allowed into the building with the patients—not even if those patients were about to receive some really shitty news. All I could do for my wife was pull up to the entrance. Cali had given me a kiss and masked up. Then she took a deep breath, exited the car, and slowly approached the hospital, looking so small and alone. I waited until the automatic doors closed behind her, knowing her life might be completely different when she walked back out, then I drove to the back corner of the CVS parking lot and waited for the doctor to call.

Twenty minutes later, Cali texted me. They were running late. An hour later, she texted again to tell me they had taken more blood, which we had not expected. It was another half hour before the doctor finally called Cali into his office.

I spent those two hours doing absolutely nothing. I didn't check my emails. I didn't look at Instagram or Facebook. I didn't play Bubble

Crush or whatever I'd been playing on the toilet that month. In fact, I didn't look at my phone at all. I didn't even listen to music or talk radio. I'm not exactly sure I was breathing. I just sat there, engine off. The car was quiet inside, and the world was quiet and gray outside—a typical winter day in Westchester County, New York.

My toes and legs got cold first. I had been sporting a sweet rotation of COVID sweatpants in recent months, and they weren't the warmest, so I eventually started the engine. *This is what it must feel like to wait for a verdict in court.*

Scenarios played out in my head.

I imagined that maybe the call wouldn't be so bad. I pictured Cali sitting in the small office chair, dwarfed by the doctor's giant mahogany desk; the good doctor's various diplomas garnishing the walls, offset by photos of his spelunking trip in Sri Lanka and stingray encounter in Bali. He'd reach for the Levitra pen he had gotten from a flirtatious pharmaceutical rep who scored him Rangers tickets last year, then say, "Great news! The biopsy was negative. We still don't know why Cali lost forty-five pounds and feels like shit all the time, but it's not cancer."

We would drive home after that, relieved, but already back to our normal ways.

"You have to take the garbage out tonight," Cali would say.

"I know, Cali," I'd respond. "It's Wednesday. The garbage goes out on Wednesday night."

"Yes, but you forget, so I'm just saying."

"I forgot once, three months ago. I do not forget all the—"

"It was two months."

"Please don't interrupt me. You always interrupt me. I'll take care of it."

Pause.

"I do not *always* interrupt you."

And so forth.

In the span of two minutes, all our worries would be forgotten. Replaced with new ones, but certainly less important. I wanted that normalcy back so badly, but I could do without the old arguments. I promised myself that if everything turned out okay, I would never let us go back to that bullshit, married-couple bickering.

What if the call wasn't good news?

The doctor would say, "It's cancer, and it's angry, my friends. It has spread aggressively while we've been doing test after test. If only we'd caught it a year ago. It's everywhere except for Cali's left eyelid. She has two weeks."

I was physically shaking that thought out of my head when my phone rang. I jumped but then answered right away, and the audio clicked through to my car speakers.

"Gregg? It's Doctor Hopewell. I'm here with Cali. Can you hear me?"

I could hear him, and I could hear Cali offer a timid "hello" in the background.

"I'm sorry the results took so long," the doctor began. "We weren't getting a concrete outcome from our lab, so we sent the sample off to Yale Labs. The pathologist there, Dr. Hemoglobin, is excellent. He was the captain of his crew team and graduated magna cum laude from Harvard. Grows his own vegetables. Very interesting fellow."

That wasn't exactly what he said, but I was on edge. The doc was beating around the bush while giving me the life story of a Yale Lab pathologist, and the suspense was killing me. *It could actually be killing my wife, with something wicked destroying her insides as each minute ticks by,* I thought.

I huffed out angrily, seeing my breath in the car. "Doc, get to the fucking point. We've screwed around for a year, leading up to this biopsy. Then we waited two weeks in horrible suspense for the results. *Then* you kept Cali waiting two hours today because you were, what, online, looking for a new boat? You won't let me in the office to hold her hand, and now you're telling me about this goddamn pathologist? I'm gonna come in there and beat you with your own nine iron."

I didn't say any of that.

I just leaned forward and adjusted the heat.

Dr. Hopewell got to the point. "Cali has stage 3S B-cell non-Hodgkin's lymphoma."

I stopped breathing.

He continued. "For lymphoma, stage 1 is neck only. Stage 2 is neck and chest. Stage 3 means that it appears above *and* below the diaphragm and also includes the pelvic region."

Pelvic region. I would've had jokes in any other situation.

He continued. "B-cell is the type of cell affected. The 'S' means that it is also in the spleen. We know that the cancer isn't in your bone marrow, because we already did that biopsy when we were trying to figure things out. Do you have any questions so far?"

I didn't have any questions so far.

Cali had a question. "Am I going to die?" she asked meekly.

The doctor paused.

I swallowed audibly.

"There is a high prognostic index. The response to treatment is eighty-five to ninety percent. There are many highly effective treatments for lymphoma that have developed in the last few decades."

I began to lose focus. The outside world faded to a gray blur. It was too much information to process while simultaneously accepting the news that my wife had cancer. Dr. Hopewell went on about something called "R-CHOP," which was an acronym for the medications they would administer during chemotherapy. He began to break down what R-CHOP stood for, and that was when my head really started spinning. He spelled out all those letters like we were little kids, and it reminded me of a certain show from my childhood.

★ ★ ★

Interior Gert and Bernie's apartment; dimly lit; gray walls. Are we in the bedroom? Living room? No one knows. Gert has already told Bernie he, Gert, has cancer and now explains the R-CHOP treatment. Bernie holds Gert's hand tenderly, nodding occasionally.

GERT

R is for rituximab, which is an antibody that targets B-cells. It is a protein. There is always

a chance of a terrible reaction, which they call
"rigors." That's why they will give it to me slowly,
over many hours. It will give me chills and fevers,
so I'll be taking lots of other meds to counteract
the symptoms.

Bernie gulps and imagines what Gert will have to endure; pictures
Gert without that cute tuft of hair at the top of his cone-shaped,
yellow head, without that adorable monobrow Bernie loves. A tear
runs down Bernie's cheek, beading up on his orange felt face.

GERT (excitedly)
That's just the first day of chemo! The next
day is sponsored by the letters C, H, and O!
That stands for a chemo cocktail made up of
cyclophosphamide, hydroxydaunomycin, and
Oncovin, which you may know as vincristine
sulfate. This mixture will hopefully kill the
bad cells. It will also kill the good ones, though,
because it is basically poison. But with any luck,
my good cells will grow back, and the bad ones
will stay dead.

Bernie stands silently, swaying, perhaps about to faint. He is
flashing back on a life spent with Gert—the good times and the
bad. The unspoken feelings, the sickening regret about ever
being cruel to his one true life partner, a wish that he could do it
all over again—but the right way this time. He even offers a short
prayer to a god in whom he doesn't even believe.

GERT
The third day is brought to you by the letter P!
P is for prednisone, which will help replace the
white blood cells that are killed by the chemicals.
There are so many crazy side effects from
prednisone!

Bernie sighs, wistfully glancing at the photo hanging on the wall of him and Gert. It is the only colorful item in the otherwise gray room.

GERT
That week of chemo plus two weeks of rest is considered one cycle. I must do six of those cycles.

Sir Counts a Lot enters, wearing a stethoscope and lab coat. The doctor's outfit covering his usual cape has not been explained, and it is not clear if he has been hiding in the apartment this entire time or if he came in through the front door.

SIR COUNTS A LOT (Transylvanian accent)
Each cycle is three! Three weeks! Then we do it over again! Six times! Yes, six cycles of three weeks comes to eighteen weeks! Ha ha ha ha!

On screen, the number eighteen flashes. It is green because that is the color of the day, which has been explained earlier in the episode. Eighteen seems a little high for a number of the day, but just go with it.

SIR COUNTS A LOT
Eighteen weeks! With some testing in between, this will take five long, terrible months! Ha ha ha ha ha.

The count vanishes in a puff of smoke. A bat is visible, flying away as the smoke clears. A pile of doctor's clothing remains.

BERNIE (close-up)
I ... I love you, Gert ....

★★★

It would have been a riveting episode.

CHAPTER 2
Paging Dr. House

Back together in the car, I held Cali for a while. When we stopped crying, we tried to look on the bright side.

"I've been through three pregnancies and three C-sections," Cali said. "I can do this. Imagine if it was *you*."

"At least he didn't call you in and tell you to get your affairs in order," I answered. "He was very optimistic."

"Maybe it's good that Hunter and Alix are away at college, and Ella is busy with high school. It will keep their minds off this."

"If you lose your hair, I'll buy you a thousand wigs."

"I just wish I had insisted that they do the biopsy earlier."

The biopsy. Earlier.

I couldn't remember exactly how it had all gone down, but in my perpetually hazy memory, Cali felt like shit for a year and then, one day, realized she was down forty-five pounds. She marched around the bedroom in her bra and panties one night, mugging it up as I lay in bed. "Look at me! Hubba-hubba! I am *so* sexy!"

She flexed and made muscles like an old-timey carnival strongman. The kind with a twirly moustache. It actually was not sexy, but it was funny. Maybe I got a *little* turned on. I mean, she did look great. And I do love carnival strongmen.

"Did you ever think you'd have *this* again? Look at these! They got so small!" She'd unfastened her bra and flashed me, shaking her newly tiny boobs like a vaudeville flapper from the twenties. Also not super sexy … but hey.

Later, we lay there sweating after making love twice. Cali was exhausted and fully satisfied. I was smoking a cigarette in a very macho way. Fine, that didn't happen. I'm pretty sure I just watched a horror movie and ignored her.

But later, we tried to figure out what was going on. Cali had been watching herself but hardly exercising or eating incredibly healthy— not enough to justify losing forty-five pounds. I had begun to notice, when Cali wasn't swaggering half naked around our bedroom, that she was walking kind of funny, like, hunched over a bit and limping. And she was always in some kind of pain or discomfort.

Various doctor's visits ensued in an effort to figure it all out. Cali saw so many different doctors that at one point, the health insurance company called and offered us a caseworker. We must have set off a code red in their system based on all the money they were shelling out. Or they were just really concerned about Cali's well-being. That must have been it. We declined the caseworker, but still, no one could figure out what the hell was happening. We needed Dr. House, George Clooney, plus Dr. McDreamy and everyone else from *Grey's Anatomy* at a time like this.

At one point, Dr. Hopewell, who was leading the charge, noticed a pattern of iron deficiency in Cali's blood test results. He prescribed ten weeks of iron infusions.

"What the fuck is an iron infusion?" I asked one night. I was thinking of pineapple-infused vodka, which is delicious, by the way.

"I go to the hospital where they do chemotherapy, but instead of chemo, they drip iron into my blood through an IV."

I was skeptical. It sounded like some voodoo bullshit.

After the first treatment, Cali came home looking forlorn. I asked what was wrong. "The treatment was fine, but it's so sad seeing all of those poor people going through chemo. I look at them and think, 'My God, we take so much for granted.'"

I mumbled something about it all being relative. If my Wi-Fi was spotty, then I was entitled to be upset.

Cali looked at me in a way that said, *You're so funny.* On second thought, maybe it was, *Why on Earth did I marry you?*

"I'm serious," she said. "The people working there are saints. I can't believe I was nervous about getting an iron infusion. Those nurses are surrounded by death and suffering, but they were still so nice to me."

After the fourth or fifth treatment, Cali came home like she'd been shot out of a cannon. She had so much energy, that I began to think we were actually onto something. Maybe her problems were all due to a chemical imbalance in her blood, and all Cali had needed was iron. I envisioned an amazing future of steak and other assorted meats for dinner.

After round eight, though, Cali's iron levels dropped off again. Her ailments were still a mystery, and she felt worse than ever. She eventually finished the infusions, but we still hadn't found the solution.

Or the problem.

A few weeks later, Cali attended her routine annual gynecological appointment. I had been working from home since the previous March during the pandemic. After Cali kissed me goodbye and headed out, I imagined her in the examining room. I've never been to a gynecologist, so I was picturing her with her legs up in stirrups surrounded by latex-clad nurses with shiny metal forceps.

Sorry, I'm an idiot.

Anyway, during that visit, the doctor felt swelling in Cali's pelvic region, which was not a good thing, like swelling in *my* pelvic region would be. They did an ultrasound and then ordered a CAT scan.

As the date approached for the CAT scan, Cali grew nervous. "I'm dying," she said to me one night.

"What? I'm reading, Cali."

"I'm dying. I'm telling you. They're going to do this CAT scan and find something awful."

I'd like to say that, in that moment, I set aside my iPad and held Cali, staring deeply into her beautiful green eyes and comforted her, saying everything would be okay.

"Cali," I said, rereading the same sentence for the third time. "You are not fucking dying. Please stop."

Then we went to bed.

What a prince.

After ten days, which I'd spent diffusing Cali's certainty that something terrible was happening, the doctor called with the results of the CAT scan. Cali's lymph nodes were enlarged. So was her spleen. Also, she had a cyst on her ovary.

"That sounds … not good," I hypothesized scientifically.

Cali concurred with my analysis. "No."

"What the fuck is a spleen, anyway?" I asked the universe.

That was when things really started happening. *Boom*, the doc ordered a needle biopsy of one of Cali's lymph nodes. The biopsy was performed by a *robot*. The robot used a needle to extract part of Cali's lymph node so they could send it out for testing. I was glad we were taking action but was somewhat uneasy since I hadn't been informed there were now robot surgeons. I wondered what other occupations had been replaced by robots and could only hope director of sales for a cosmetic packaging company was not one of them.

We endured an excruciating two-week wait for the results of the needle biopsy. Two nerve-wracking weeks of wondering what we would learn. By now, I was concerned. Shit was getting real. Things inside Cali were not the size they were supposed to be. Parts were enlarged. Organs were involved—spleens even.

I'd lost my ability to casually dismiss Cali's concerns, and I began to wonder what exactly was happening to my wife. I looked up her maladies online and didn't make it past the first page of horrors. If you ever have something bothering you, don't search for it online. Go to a doctor.

Also, don't look up blue waffle. Just a PSA while I have you.

Finally, we had an appointment to receive the results of the robot needle biopsy. I joined on speakerphone, mildly wondering if the robot would be on the call. I was in the CVS parking lot across from the hospital, which I would eventually get to know intimately.

Prior to this, I had looked up Dr. Hopewell online to see if there were any reviews, and that was a mistake too. Everyone had really nice things to say, but the photo of him threw me off. Dude looked just like Ed Sheeran. This explains why I imagined the doctor holding a guitar when he told us that the results were inconclusive.

He explained, "You see, a lymph node is not a solid structure, so getting some of it to pass into a needle is somewhat difficult. It is not a very accurate test."

I began to suspect we were being taken for a ride. First iron infusions, and now this. Why had we just wasted all that time and energy on an inaccurate robot needle test?

The doctor added, "However, from what we can tell, the results are negative."

I pulled out of the CVS and drove up to the hospital. Cali came outside ecstatic. "I don't have cancer!" she exclaimed as she got in the car.

On our way home, Cali immediately called her parents to tell them the news. Then she called her sister, Shari. Then she called her brother, Sean, and texted her friends. Everyone thought it was wonderful news. We barely said a word to each other on the drive home while Cali broadcasted to the universe.

But as I drove, I began to wonder. *How much lymph node juice did that robot get, if any? And how do you base your diagnosis on a faulty test? Also, is there a Taco Bell on the way home?*

★ ★ ★

"I'd like to try another approach."

Cali had returned to Dr. Hopewell's office for a follow-up visit. I was back in the CVS parking lot on speakerphone, wondering if CVS security had my picture on a wall somewhere. Dr. Sheeran—er, Hopewell—was recapping that he wanted to take more blood, do more tests, and embark on the next steps in our journey to figure out what was troubling Cali since she *didn't have cancer.*

The doc further explained why the needle biopsy done by those "wascally wobots" had been so inaccurate. Or unreliable. Or why a negative result wasn't exactly 100 percent. It wasn't totally clear what he was saying as he was talking in circles a bit. The doc seemed to be hedging his bets, but the bottom line was "they" weren't even sure they'd gotten any of the lymph node material. Which, to me, meant the test of the lymph node might be negative, but it also might not be a test of the lymph node. It was kind of like doing a preflight maintenance check on a Boeing 747 and clearing it for wheels up, but you're not sure if you checked the right plane. Or if it even was a plane. Or if you actually work at the airport.

Also, there was a decent chance those robot surgeons had decided we humans were the virus, and this was Phase One of their plans to eradicate us.

The doctor felt strongly that we should go ahead and surgically remove a lymph node to send it out for testing. This was based on the inaccuracy of the needle biopsy and the fact that Cali's gynecologist had recently felt an enlarged node in the pelvic region.

I've spent some time in the pelvic region. So relaxing. A little humid though.

All of this was "just to rule everything out." That was how the doctor put it.

I'd pictured Lieutenant Frank Drebin from *The Naked Gun* in front of an exploding fireworks factory, waving his arms. *Keep moving, folks. Nothing to see here.*

Also, that meddling gyno had noticed a cyst on one of Cali's favorite ovaries. So, while they were in there, they could offer us a two-for-one and remove that as well.

Anything else? Well, since you asked, how about we go ahead and perform a full hysterectomy on your wife to avoid any other unforeseen problems in the future?

I'd imagined a giant surgical ice cream scooper relieving Cali of all those pesky organs. *What would Baskin-Robbins name that flavor?* I wondered.

That night, Cali and I were binge-watching *Deadwood* in bed. I looked over and noticed she was crying. It was not a sad moment in the program, although Timothy Olyphant is an excellent actor. I quickly recalled from the official husband handbook that crying was a pause-the-show situation, so I paused the show and asked Cali what was wrong.

"I'm not going to be a … woman anymore," she sobbed, talking about her impending hysterectomy.

Shit. That was rather heavy, and I hadn't thought about it.

Cali'd had her period almost every month since she was twelve, so at fifty-two years old, that was … carry the two … well, *a lot* of periods. She had also made three amazing babies with those lovely lady parts. Plus, you know, I liked the whole set up down there too.

I began to understand that having a hysterectomy was much more significant than removing, say, a mole. There was no emotional attachment to a mole. You couldn't imagine its purpose. You don't romanticize that time your mole created life or was the center of your romantic relationship.

Plus, there were the hormonal changes to consider.

What would that be like? I wondered, shuddering. *Yikes.*

I told Cali I would love her no matter what, even if they gave her a penis, which I immediately wished I could take back. But really, I meant I'd be there for her no matter what. This was where the rubber met the road, and I had made Cali a promise. *In sickness and in health. Right?*

I hit play after comforting her, and we went back to watching filthy prostitutes treat their bodies like storefronts.

★ ★ ★

Due to COVID, they didn't let me into the hospital for the surgery to remove the lymph node and the uterus and the ovaries and the things. So, after dropping Cali off at the hospital very early, I went home. I ate breakfast and tried to work but was mostly waiting for the next text from Cali.

8:00 a.m.
Prev surgery running late, so not starting at 9:30. More like 11

11:00 a.m.
No word from surgeon yet so def not starting at 11

12:00 p.m.
Prev surgery done now so hopefully soon

2:00 p.m.
No sign of him yet hopefully soon

3:00 p.m.
OK they're going to take me soon

This poor woman had been alone and lying around nervously for eight hours before they took her in for surgery. My God.

Ella and I were having dinner at home that evening when my cell rang. It was Dr. Guntz, the surgeon. *Guntz*. What a name.

I had never met him. Neither had Cali, really. When he finally showed up that day, he'd introduced himself and then dived right in. It was the fastest anyone had ever gotten into Cali's pants. Hopefully.

Anyway, it quickly became apparent that Guntz had a less-than-warm demeanor, if you know what I mean. If you don't know what I mean, I'll clarify: He was a giant dick.

"The surgery was successful. I took a lymph node for testing and performed a full hysterectomy. The patient is in recovery for the next two hours. The patient will stay here overnight. There was a lot of swelling of the lymph nodes and the spleen. Any questions?"

"Yes, Doctor, my wife's name is Cali, and she is a fellow human. Please don't refer to her as 'the patient' again, or I will shatter your nose." I didn't say that, yet it all felt so clinical and brief that I did feel compelled to ask *something*. "Can you clarify what you mean by 'a lot of swelling'?"

"Well," Dr. Delightful said. "The presurgical notes from the CAT scan said 'minor swelling.' I wouldn't call what I saw 'minor'!" He seemed amused by the intricacies of this wacky English language and the various ways someone could describe the swollen insides of my wife.

I hung up, not exactly feeling reassured. I thought this surgery and subsequent biopsy was just to *rule everything out*. Why did Guntz say that about the swelling? More importantly, *why* was there so much swelling?

Fast-forward two weeks, and we're in the car processing the lymphoma bomb Dr. Hopewell just dropped on us.

CHAPTER 3
Meet the Parents

We drove straight from the hospital to Cali's parents' house. She wanted to give them the news in person, naturally.

Cali's parents live in Hidden Hills, six miles from our house, in an inexplicably massive 2,500-unit townhouse community. There are pools, tennis courts, a golf course, and a clubhouse, just like a Floridian retirement community. But it is not adults only. And it is not in Florida. I don't know who built this place or why, but it exists. Cali's folks moved here from Brooklyn when we began spawning offspring, so it was very convenient. It was the perfect location between us in Somers and Cali's sister Shari's family in Armonk. Cali's brother and his family live in Manhattan.

I got out of the car and walked around to help Cali out. It was icy, and I didn't want her to slip. Plus, I figured her parents were looking out the window, and sadly, I was still trying to score brownie points after all these years. We walked carefully up the walkway, bracing ourselves against a slip on the ice and for the conversation that was about to take place. Cali's Dad opened the front door as we approached.

★★★

There's a scene in Quentin Tarantino's *Reservoir Dogs* when Tim Roth's undercover cop, Freddy, is asked by his partner to describe Joe, the crime boss.

FREDDY

You remember the Fantastic Four?

HOLDAWAY

Yeah, with that invisible bitch, "Flame On!" and that shit?

FREDDY

The Thing; motherfucker looks like The Thing.

I always think of that scene when I describe Cali's father, "Big Al" Leibowitz. Big Al was never a baby. He'd emerged from his mother a fully grown, strapping teenager and immediately began playing football for New Utrecht High School in Brooklyn. That's the school in the opening credits of *Welcome Back, Kotter*, by the way. He then went on to play at the University of New Mexico. His teammates there thought he was a sheriff because of the giant gold badge hanging from his neck. It was a Jewish star, but they had never seen one before.

Back home after college, Big Al became a physical education teacher and then the head football coach at his alma mater, New Utrecht. While teaching and coaching, Al held several other jobs. I've heard that Coach—as all his former players still call him—would come home for dinner, eat with the family, and then go right back out to work at a local college or YMCA. Cali never has any stories about the things they couldn't afford. Big Al provided.

Ultimately, he became the principal of New Utrecht and later took the position of New York City Football Commissioner. His former players are in their seventies, which makes no sense because Al is in his seventies. Was he five years old when he coached them? It's possible. What I do know is that generations of Brooklynites worship him.

When they approach me, they always ask, "You Big Al's son-in-law?"

"Yes, I am," I respond.

"Coach is a great man. When I was young, I didn't have parents. My sister and I lived in a nest. One day, your father-in-law, he grabs me by the neck and says, 'You and your sister live in the equipment shed now.' Every day before school started, your father-in-law would walk around back, unlock the shed, and regurgitate a little of his breakfast into our mouths. He fed us that way for four years. He taught me how to play football and then threatened Joe Paterno until he accepted me on full scholarship at Penn State. I owe that motherfucker my *life*."

There have been many stories like this.

Having helped so many local families, Big Al might have been somewhat "connected" over the years, if you know what I mean.

"I'm going to tell everybody who walks in this building that in apartment 2R, Janice Rossi is nothing but a *whore*!"

Sorry, I am compelled to reference *Goodfellas* when anyone mentions the Mafia. Even if that someone is me.

Anyway, later, when Big Al retired, he did not *actually* retire. He became the director of Tyler Hill Camp in Pennsylvania, where he had previously run the waterfront every summer and gained the moniker Big Al due to his large personality ... and possibly his girth. Along with his wife, Arlene, Big Al ran that summer camp of over five hundred kids for almost fifteen years.

Before he had his first grandchild and quit smoking cold turkey *that exact day*, Big Al had enjoyed Middleton's Black & Mild pipe tobacco cigarillos. They are long and thin cigars with a plastic tip and an unmistakable *stank*. When he was done with one, he would jam the smoldering butt into the nearest tree. If you needed to find him up at camp, you could follow the plastic mouthpieces, like the world's most disturbing breadcrumb trail. If there wasn't a tree nearby, he may have just eaten the butts. Unconfirmed.

After running the camp, Al retired again in 2005, but again, he didn't actually retire. Not really. He consulted at another summer camp for two years with Arlene. *Then* he retired but later grew his local legend here in Westchester when he became assistant football coach at Byram Hills High School, where my nephew Hayden played. Also, final note, Al is made of rock. His calves are still the size of boulders. He has thick rhino skin and no neck.

I tell you this so you understand. This man has always been large and in charge. He has always been revered, feared, and respected. He has always been obeyed, without question, in every position of authority he held. As a result, maybe he's had some difficulty adjusting to life up in the suburbs where he is no longer the "mayor of Brooklyn." His grown children and their independently minded spouses make their own decisions. Knowing this, maybe that's why I give him a pass when he tells me my lawn looks a little "off," or I should really reseal my driveway this spring, even though I already fucking knew that. Maybe I let him give advice to my kids, even if it mostly applies to a kid from the fifties who got beat up after a stickball game. My kids understand too.

In all fairness, I should also say Al has softened a bit. He saw his daughters grow up and become women. Watched them marry idiots. He has amazing grandchildren. Saw those grandchildren grow slightly older and become idiots. He watched his son, Sean, create an amazing family too, while dealing with some of life's fun curveballs. And he outlived a few people he loved dearly. All of it humbled him a little. *A little.*

My mother-in-law, Arlene, may as well be the female version of my father-in-law, although she is significantly better looking. She, too, is a no-nonsense badass. Her father died when she was young. She and her two brothers lived in a small apartment with their mother and some aunts and maybe some other characters. I don't know the actual details, but in the stories I've heard, it sounded crowded. Who knows how they survived, but let me put it this way: The world did not beat Arlene—and neither will you.

Arlene might not have *kvelled* over me the way I'd always imagined my future mother-in-law would. In fact, walking into her townhouse that awful February day, I was pretty sure I was about to have my first real conversation with her in twenty-three years. Just kidding ...

mostly. Arlene tolerates me, but the woman *loves* her children. She *lives* for her children and her grandchildren.

Cali and her mother talk on the phone all the time. And then, they talk on the phone some more. In between, Arlene talks on the phone with Cali's older sister, Shari. They tell each other things they already just told each other, and sometimes the sisters will tell Arlene things the other sister just told her. Cali will talk on the phone with her mother, go pick her mother up for nails and lunch, and then get home and call her mother to chat.

And they can talk about anything in great detail. I once heard Cali describe her trip through the supermarket to her mother for *an hour*. That was longer than she'd actually been in the supermarket. Also, *nothing happened* at the supermarket.

When Cali says goodbye to her mom on the phone, I don't suddenly perk up because I am about to get my wife back. That first goodbye means nothing because one of them will realize they forgot to tell the other something, and it all starts back up again. There will be at least five more false goodbyes before it ends. This happens in person too, which is tough for me because I generally want to leave wherever I am right away, and they make it difficult.

Also, Cali's mother knows everything. I don't mean that sarcastically, like she *thinks* she knows everything. Arlene Leibowitz *actually knows everything*. Early on, when the kids were little, Arlene would know when something was off.

"She has thrush," she would state unequivocally after staring at the baby's tongue.

"Make sure they check his growth plate on the X-ray." *Growth plate? That's a thing?*

"Give her two teaspoons of honey but mix in one drop of hydrogen peroxide."

She didn't really say that last one, so don't try it at home.

It was intimidating for me as a young lad and new father. I didn't have a goddamn clue about being married or owning a home, much less taking care of babies. But I was too stubborn and insecure to gracefully accept Arlene's assistance. Early on, she unintentionally served as a constant reminder to me that I didn't know jack shit. In my defense, she may not have "observed boundaries" or "cared what I thought" or "known that I existed." So, we silently butted heads a bit in the early days, and not so silently once or twice. But it's all good now ... I think.

Yes, I like to think we grew to respect each other over the years. I could be wrong. I respect them, at least. Both of Cali's parents.

The main reason I have grown to love and respect my tough, headstrong, boundary-neutral in-laws is because of their generosity. They are generous with their time and presence, they are generous financially, and they are generous with their love. They will do absolutely anything for their kids and grandkids. They'll kill for them. Trust me, Big Al has offered. He knows a few guys, just say the word. They've taken this crazy family of sixteen on several Caribbean vacations. They always insist on paying for dinner, buying gifts, and giving the kids money before they head off to school, a trip, the bathroom. They will show up anywhere, anytime, no matter what. They've been to their grandchildren's recitals, sporting events, performances, graduations, presentations, and bowel movements. If the event allows guests, they are there. And, if the event doesn't allow guests, they are there anyway. Hardly any social life, if any. All about the family.

Sometimes, I imagine Al and Arlene getting home and just shutting down like the grandparents in *Weird Science*. Standing frozen in the closet until the next dance recital or soccer game, only to then reanimate and head back out.

So, occasionally it gets annoying for a dummy like me. But then again, I am easily irritated and probably a little jealous since my parents live in Florida. You must admit though. Their dedication is impressive.

★ ★ ★

There we were. Arlene, Cali, Big Al, and yours truly sitting at the round kitchen table in Hidden Hills Unit 2311M. We had filled them in on the details of Cali's diagnosis. Arlene cried off and on, and it was a bit shocking to see her sans makeup and coiffure. Al wouldn't make eye contact and was fidgeting with something in his hands—nope, there was nothing in his hands—when he suddenly got up and walked out of the room. A few minutes later, he called for me to come help him figure something out on his computer. I excused myself and went in to his office/guest room.

"See this screen here?" he pointed at the screen with his meaty index finger.

I saw the screen there, and I told him so.

"This screen usually has a bunch of things on it, but now it doesn't."

I sat down and had a look. There was a window on the screen with three app icons. There were two dots at the bottom. The dot on the right was white, and the one on the left was dark. He was on Page Two. He had unknowingly turned the page. He was used to seeing Page One with all the other apps, not this second page with only the last three.

He hovered close to my shoulder, smelling like Old Spice, breathing heavily.

I swiped the mouse to get back to Page One.

"There it is," he told me, pointing again.

"Should be good now," I told him.

I stood up. He remained in place, still looking at the computer. We were awkwardly close to each other and silent for a moment. I wanted to put my hand on his giant shoulder and tell him I had this situation under control. He needn't feel powerless as his baby girl was attacked from the inside out by cancer. I wanted to tell him I was going to be there for Cali, no matter what. I loved his daughter and would do anything to protect her from pain or suffering, and I would make sure she felt safe and loved at all times.

"Okay … well," I said.

"Yep, thanks for the help with that," he said back.

We went back into the kitchen.

CHAPTER 4

The Little Fockers

I had to tell the kids. Our youngest, Ella, was still at high school, so I had to wait. My son, Hunter, a junior at Ohio State, and my other daughter, Alix, a sophomore at Tulane, were both away at school, having the best shitty experience they possibly could while attending college during the wonderful age of COVID.

I video-chatted with Hunter first.

"What's up, Padre?" he greeted me cheerfully. He likes to call me "Padre."

Hunter's room in his frat house was barely lit by a blue LED strip. I could just make out the silhouette of his dark-brown hair, which he had been growing out during quarantine and was wild. He looked like a young Einstein. He was shirtless and clearly still in bed. It was 1 p.m.

I told him the news without beating around the bush or mincing words. "Mom got the results of her biopsy today. She has lymphoma."

"What's that?" Still somewhat upbeat.

"It's cancer."

The smile dropped from his face. His phone wobbled slightly, swaying as he absorbed what I told him. Did I catch a glimpse of a huge bong on the side table? Nah, it must have been a stack of textbooks; it was hard to see. Even in the dark-blue light, I could make out splotches forming around his eyes. He was crying now.

The call with Alix was worse. She cried harder, down there in New Orleans, and it was harder for me to console her. I suddenly felt like everything I said sounded phony. I didn't know everything would be okay. I didn't know her mom would be just fine. I didn't know anything. But I explained the situation and the prognosis and then listed all the other things I could think of that would make her look on the bright side.

"I want to come home," she said.

"I don't think you can, Freckles." I call her "Freckles" because she has freckles. I'm creative like that. "Mom has to be really careful now not to catch anything, especially COVID. Her immune system is going to take a beating."

"I'll stay at Aunt Shari's."

I explained why that wouldn't make any sense. Alix still wouldn't be able to hug her mom or spend time with her if she were here; therefore, it wasn't worth leaving college. Plus, Cali and I had spoken about this. It was very important to us both that the kids didn't let this turn their lives upside-down. We wanted them to continue to enjoy college as much as possible, despite how limited that experience already was. Should I say "due to COVID" again? Nah, you get it.

"Listen," I said to Alix. "I've got this. She has the best care, and all of us here will be looking after her. Plus, I'm working from home right now, which is good timing."

"I don't care, I want to come home."

I told her we'd see.

Next up: Ella.

I waited anxiously at the front window, pacing a little. Our Bengal cats, Keanu and Loki, sat stoically, following me carefully with their eyes. Their heads moved back and forth as I walked from window to front door and back to window, peering out and down the street. Their human was acting strangely, and they were not going to miss the show.

Cali was upstairs, as I requested, because I wanted to speak to Ella alone first when she got home from school. The chaos of the two of us trying to explain things to our youngest child would surely end in bickering, and I wanted to avoid that. I'd give Ella a clear message, let her digest the information, and then she could go talk with Cali.

That's the right way. *Or is it?* I second-guessed myself.

Maybe Cali should speak to Ella alone, and I was being self-serving by wanting to tell her myself. Or maybe we should tell her together, showing a united front and thus signaling everything would be okay. Surely, we could manage that without screwing it up. I didn't know. I suddenly felt I didn't know *anything*, really. I never learned how to balance a checkbook. How the fuck was I supposed to know what to do in *this* situation?

That day, school ended at 1:20 p.m. The schedule was all over the place this year—say it with me—*due to COVID*. Some days, Ella was home, fully taking her classes online. Other days, she was at school in person until 1:40 p.m. *Other* days, she got home just after 10 a.m., after only being at school for two or three hours. I never knew when she would be home or not, and, of course, only Cali had the schedule memorized. Only Cali woke up at 6 a.m. to submit the mandatory online COVID screening form each morning and to make sure Ella was awake.

One morning, a few months back, I'd been working from home as usual, and Cali was headed out. She was going grocery shopping.

"Where's Ella?" I asked before Cali left. I was asking for a reason.

"At school," Cali said as she walked out the door.

I was actually alone in my own home. It had been a while. So, let's just say I had some "alone" time.

Ten minutes later, I'd gone back to work, a huge weight lifted off my balls ... er, I mean, shoulders. I heard a door slam upstairs and jumped, ready to fight any intruders to my own quick death. Ella came bounding down the stairs in her workout clothes. "Done with school, Dad! Going downstairs to work out."

I almost had a heart attack.

Later that night, I told Cali what had happened. "You said Ella was at school!" I exclaimed.

"She was!"

Technically. In her room though. We'd sorted out some clear terminology after that.

Anyway, the high school was fifteen minutes from our house, at most. It was 1:45 p.m., and as I said, school ended at 1:20 p.m. Where the hell was Ella? I started pacing more rapidly, causing the cats to look at me with some mild concern. Or maybe they didn't give a shit. I watched them, envious of their tiny brains and simple lives. And their ability to lick themselves.

A car pulled into the driveway. Ella's friend had driven her home. I walked briskly from the house into the garage and hit the button, opening the garage door. Ella, looking so grown up and completely unaware of what was to come, walked up the driveway.

My little Pipsqueak isn't so little anymore, I thought, recalling another awful winter day.

★★★

It was New Year's Eve 2004. Cali and I pulled into the Connecticut townhouse community where we lived back then. It was our first night out since the Christmas Eve birth of our beautiful daughter, Ella Joy Goldman. Our third child, and she was hard-earned.

None of Cali's pregnancies had been easy, but she handled them like a champ. We'd be standing around talking to someone, and Cali would excuse herself, throw up into a garbage pail, and come back to continue the conversation. She'd also had three C-sections, each of which got tougher and tougher due to the build-up of scar tissue from each previous surgery. Things got weird during the last delivery. There was a lot of shouting and activity on the other side of the curtain while I spoke quiet, comforting words to my pale, shivering wife on our side. I don't even want to know what really happened over there.

For this reason, Cali and our Christmas Eve baby spent a few additional days in the hospital recovering. Now we were all home and getting into a nice routine with our temporary live-in baby nurse, a large and gentle Jamaican woman named Dorothy. Cali finally felt well enough physically and comfortable enough with Dorothy to go out and see a movie with me on New Year's Eve.

We went straight home after the movie. Cali hadn't wanted to go to dinner or anything else. It was hard enough for her to be away for as long as we were. Personally, I would have flown to Bali if she'd been up for it.

We entered our townhouse and got a positive report on Ella from Dorothy, who was washing bottles in the kitchen. It felt good to be in the warm safety of our rental townhouse, surrounded by a fortress of IKEA furniture we had somehow assembled without killing each other. It was snowing out, a large flaky snow that came down lazily. We took our boots off, hung up our coats, and headed down to the finished basement where Ella would be under Dorothy's care for the next two weeks. Cali was still totally hands-on but had to focus on her own recovery as well. And I was, you know, there.

After blowing kisses to our sleeping beauty, we quietly went back upstairs and stood at each of our other kids' bedroom doorways for a moment. My in-laws had watched them for us and dropped them off earlier. Sometimes, it still felt like we were playing house, but these amazing little kids were all ours. *We made them*, I often marveled. Hunter lay splayed out in his big-boy bed, sweaty, his hair a mess. Almost five, he was getting too big for his cute little truck pajamas. The pants stopped mid-shin and the sleeves mid-forearm. And Alix, asleep in her room, twenty-two months younger than her brother, lying on her side, curled up, and surrounded by stuffed animals. She was wearing a little purple Barbie nightgown.

On this New Year's Eve, even then, we recognized how lucky we were. How *blessed*, if that's your cup of tea. We headed into our bedroom and began to get changed for bed.

"Miss Cali! Miss Cali!" Dorothy suddenly yelled from downstairs. "Miss Cali, come quick!"

I ran downstairs, skipping steps at a time, with Cali close behind me.

Dorothy stood in the kitchen over the sink. Her back was to us, and she was holding something. Her head was down.

Is she blowing up a balloon? That doesn't make any sense.

She turned her head toward us. "Baby's no breathing, Miss Cali."

I stepped closer, staring in absolute horror as Dorothy bent her head back down, put her mouth over Ella's, and began to blow. I mentally deciphered the situation. For whatever reason, Ella was not breathing, and Dorothy was administering CPR. I was in shock, watching her. I imagined the police interviewing me later, notebook in hand. "So, let me get this straight. You just stood there and let this stranger give your baby CPR while you did nothing?"

I flashed forward through the rest of my life, haunted by a dead baby and the nagging certainty I could have saved her. I'd be judged by my family, resented by my wife, hated by Cali's family. I'd be racked with guilt for doing nothing in the face of adversity. And, although it appeared that Dorothy was indeed administering CPR properly, I'd be damned if it wasn't going to be me who determined whether my little girl lived or died.

I scooped Ella into my arms and yelled to Cali. "Call 9-1-1 *right now*! Tell them to send an ambulance!"

Cali was in shock. She was wide-eyed and screaming something.

I ignored her and put my mouth over Ella's tiny mouth and nose. I'd been a certified lifeguard years ago and somehow still remembered the basics of CPR. As I held Ella's little body in my arms, Cali blinked and moved to the phone on the wall. She managed to make the call and frantically gave our address. Ella's little belly puffed up each time I breathed air into her, but she remained limp and unresponsive. I blew harder, worrying I would pop her lungs—*Is that possible?*—or do some other permanent damage. But none of that mattered; I *had* to get her breathing. As I blew, I moved toward the front door and slipped my feet into my unlaced boots. Our townhouse community had a mile-long, curved, one-way road running through it, with only one entrance and one exit. I ran out the front door and down the street toward that front entrance, still giving Ella breaths, hoping I could save precious seconds by intercepting the ambulance when it pulled into the neighborhood.

It had stopped snowing. My boots sloshed through the fresh wet snow.

Cali ran behind me, screaming. "Don't let my baby die! Oh my God, don't let my baby die!"

Dorothy stood in the doorway, silhouetted by the light behind her. We hadn't said a word, but she knew what to do. Stay behind and look after the kids. Later, we learned Shari and my brother-in-law, Aaron, had come over to help.

In the ambulance, Cali rode in back with Ella and the EMTs. I rode in front, wondering if our lives were about to change forever. Would this be the night we lost our child? Would we ever forgive ourselves for going out tonight? Would Cali and I make it through this?

They got Ella breathing again in the ambulance, and we followed her on the gurney up to the NICU. It was now just after midnight, and the nurses on staff were quietly celebrating the New Year with party hats and a cake. We interrupted.

Ella spent the next three days in the NICU, and we spent those three days camped out in the waiting area. She hadn't lost oxygen to her brain long enough to do any damage. The whole thing turned out to be caused by reflux, so she was put on a special formula. The next two weeks at home, Ella was hooked to an apparatus that measured her vitals and screamed an unholy siren if anything was wrong. Or if one of the sticky tabs fell off. Or if she moved. It was a tense time.

Two weeks later, I held Ella, free of the wires and tubes. She was pink and healthy and bundled up in a blankie. I put my head to hers.

"I've got you, Pipsqueak," I whispered. "I've got you."

★★★

Now age sixteen and considerably taller, Ella stood in the cold garage, her giant backpack looking like it was going to tip her over. I suggested she take it off, but she could sense something was wrong. She could see it in my eyes. And I didn't normally meet her in the garage when she returned from school. She kept the backpack on.

I told her about her mom. As she cried, I held her for a long time, my arms wrapped awkwardly around my little Pipsqueak and her giant backpack.

CHAPTER 5
The Giant Turd

The next few days were a blur. The team at Northern Westchester Hospital had made an astounding number of appointments for Cali. This was an incredible relief, as I had envisioned us spending the next month angrily waiting to see various doctors before we could take any action while the cancer continued its possibly deadly course.

All those appointments also kept Cali busy. There was a surgical follow-up from her lymphadenectomy and hysterectomy. There was a presurgical clearance for chemo, an EKG at the cardiologist, a consult with the doctor who would install a port in her chest, a CAT scan, and finally a PET scan to determine a baseline. All were interspersed with a new round of iron infusions. There was very little time to dwell on things.

I couldn't attend any of these doctor visits because of COVID, so I drove Cali and then sat in the car in the good-old CVS parking lot. I spent some time thinking and half-heartedly answering work emails, but a lot of my energy was focused on trying not to shit myself. I know that sounds crazy, but I was sitting in a parking lot for hours at a time with no access to a bathroom. I was afraid to go into the CVS and miss an important call. Don't judge. It was a good distraction.

One night that first week, Cali asked me to put together a group text to give all her close friends the news. It seemed strange to send this grave information in a text, but there was no way I was calling each person individually, so I agreed. I was surprised at the size of the list, considering Cali and I are not very social people. In fact, some might say we are antisocial.

We moved to Somers in 2005, right after that incident with Ella, actually. We built a house so far north of New York City that, to my dismay, people told me they had "summer homes" up there. But as the house prices rose, and we were being shown million-dollar dumps closer to the city, it became apparent we were going to have to look farther north to find something we could afford. And live in.

Apparently, a lot of other people had the same idea. By 2007, the Somers population consisted of six horse farmers who had lived there forever and hundreds of young families from all over the tristate area seeking affordable and inhabitable homes. The result was a less-than-diverse melting pot of what seemed like mostly Italian and Irish. There was a sprinkling of us Jews in there too, like any great recipe that calls for a pinch of kosher salt.

Our neighborhood was called The Woodlands—aptly named because although the builders had leveled every tree and stripped every inch of topsoil, they were legally bound to preserve at least some of the surrounding woodlands. The resulting neighborhood consisted of 180 very similar homes with one identical tree in front of each and a patch of woods here and there in between.

There were new neighborhoods just like The Woodlands every few miles in Somers. All were filled with families who might have otherwise settled anywhere else but missed the boat by a few years. And, aside from the distance to the city, it was actually a nice place to live. My point being that the next fifteen-plus years in Somers were pretty fun. The town was filled with young families looking to mingle, go out to dinner, have playdates, and host book clubs, backyard barbecues, parties, and poker games.

Cali and I participated but were different than most. Maybe we were insecure and didn't completely put ourselves out there. I like to think we were *too* secure and knew exactly who we did and did not want to spend our time with. Either way, we were perfectly happy sitting home on a Friday night, playing with the kids while ordering in and hanging out. In addition, my actual job required quite a lot of entertaining and socializing, so it was the last thing I wanted to do in my free time. Plus, Cali's family was so close that any special occasion—like Fourth of July, New Year's Eve, heck, Groundhog Day—was spent together, thus not affording us the opportunity to really mix it up. We liked it that way though.

And so, we became acquaintances of many and only truly friendly with few. We continued to meet people, mostly because of Cali. Lord knows I wasn't seeking anyone out. Cali would befriend people at school events, soccer practice, the bus stop, the supermarket. We entered a comfortable period of loosely socializing with many couples but avoided getting very close to most. We knew what we were missing thanks to social media, and we didn't care.

"Oh, they had that Orange Party last night," Cali said, showing me her phone. "We should have gone!" She scrolled through countless photos of what seemed like the entire population of Somers dressed in orange and cavorting drunkenly.

We looked at each other and laughed. "Nah, we're good."

The couples we became friendly with began to understand how we operated over time; mostly because we told them straight out.

"We don't like many people, but we like you guys," we would declare. It was always a big moment in our relationships.

My one buddy, Michael Y., took a while longer to understand where I was coming from.

One evening, he texted me, Passing by your house, wanna come out and take a walk?

I took a personal inventory. My sweats were already on after a long day working in the city. I was lying on the couch with my phone in hand and a beer balanced on my stomach. The kids were playing on the floor.

Nah, I'm good, thx, I typed.

It finally came to a head one Tuesday night.

Yo, beers? read the text from Michael.

My family had just finished eating dinner together, which was always very important to us, and now we were sitting around the living room on our various devices. The girls were practicing a new dance and would soon perform it in front of the fireplace. And I mentioned it was Tuesday, right?

Nah, I'm good thx, I typed.

Dude, I give up, he wrote hastily, having been politely turned down by me one too many times.

The next time I saw Mr. Y., I explained. "Look, man, I like hanging with you. I'm not blowing you off. But when I get home from work, all I want to do is veg out and chill with my family, so don't take it personally. We good?"

I should mention I spent almost four hours a day in the car, heading to and from the city, while Michael worked at home. That fucker probably couldn't *wait* to get out of his house.

So we formed an understanding with Michael and his wife Brenda just like we did with anyone else who enjoyed our company. If you wanted to hang with Cali and Gregg, you had to accept our flaky quirks. We knew the risk: People would eventually get fed up with us, and we'd be completely alone, but we were okay with that.

We are also prone to canceling at the last minute, which I admit is pretty shitty. But we are upfront about that too. We'll make plans, and someone will say they are looking forward to it.

We'll say, "Yeah, if we don't cancel on you, it'll be fun."

This all resulted, though, in a down-to-earth crew who totally understood how we rolled and knew what to expect.

I tell you this because I was pleasantly surprised when Cali gave me the list of people to contact. In spite of ourselves, we had managed to accumulate quite a number of friends—or Cali had. And I was pleased with the quality as well. If our goal was to never spend time with people we didn't like, then we had succeeded.

I sent out the awkwardly worded group text, feeling bad about the giant turd I was about to drop in everyone's lap but not knowing a better way.

Call me a terrible person, but I've never been very good at giving much of a shit about most other people. I have a crazy job where I am always taking care of customers. I have a family, which is my number-one priority. And, quite frankly, I have to take care of myself. Which, if you've seen me lately, you'd know I am not doing a great job of.

So, when I hear that so-and-so's grandmother passed away, yes, I feel bad. Yes, I wish them the best. But I am not going to a funeral for a lady I never met. Nor am I willing to give up my time to go pay a shiva call, visit a hospital, or do anything really. I go if Cali forces me—under protest—but otherwise, I stay in my bubble.

You don't have to like me. In fact, you can end our friendship over it if it means I don't have to show up, which has actually happened. Hey, I'm just being honest. I'm not saying it's right.

Also, when I hear someone is sick or has cancer, it doesn't click for me. I still feel disconnected. Maybe something is wrong with me. Who knows.

"Uncle Mitchell has prostate cancer," my mother once informed me from Florida during our weekly call.

"Oh, man. Tell him I say ... um, 'Hang in there.'"

That was it.

My awesome Uncle Mitchell: amazing memories from growing up and playing with my cousins in his house; totally love him and his whole family; the warmest guy with a huge heart—and huge prostate apparently. I didn't reach out. I didn't check in with his kids. I didn't do anything.

Hang in there.

What a sport.

So I admit I had low expectations after I texted the news about Cali. Yet, one actual minute after hitting send, the most heartfelt and loving messages began flowing in, and I was sincerely moved. I read each one to Cali. Once they communicated their shock and sorrow, her friends offered encouragement and support.

She's a warrior! She will crush this!

We all love her so much!

She has the most amazing family and friends who love her so much. She's got this!

I'm paraphrasing, but it was an outpouring of love expressed in such a genuine way that we both got choked up message after message.

It made me want to be better.

CHAPTER 6
A Second Opinion, Technically

They put a port in Cali's chest on Monday, March 1. It was a surgical procedure, but in and out the same day. Cali said they knocked her out with the same medication Michael Jackson had been addicted to—propofol. She said it is commonly used in outpatient surgery, like when you get a colonoscopy. I told her I hoped they hadn't accidentally put the port up her ass.

Colonoscopy jokes ….

So anyway, they installed this contraption under the skin of her upper right chest. Now they could plug right into Cali's port for chemo and the administration of other drugs, instead of poking holes in her arm every time for an IV.

The port protruded from under her skin, like a baby alien trying to escape. There was a hard tube running from the port up her neck that bulged out slightly and another tube running down to her heart. The day she got it, she asked if I wanted to touch it, and I said no. Then I touched it, and it freaked me out. I felt a dull ache right in my balls.

I'm no shrinking violet. I bow and rifle hunt and field dress my own deer. I've been shoulder-deep inside said deer while field dressing. I watch tons of horror movies because I'm a freak and find them relaxing. I even had to change the packing in Cali's still-open c-section incision for a month after Alix was born, and it hadn't bothered me much. I don't get squeamish easily. But that port in Cali's chest freaked me out.

There's only one way I can describe it: unnatural.

Three days after the port installation, I was working in my home office when our fancy-ass doorbell signaled movement in front of the house. I had been ignoring these alerts since it seemed we lately had packages delivered almost hourly. There was often a FedEx or UPS truck in the driveway, and I was tired of checking the camera because it only reminded me of how much money we were spending. Cancer was not slowing my wife down when it came to online shopping. In fact, cancer provided a whole new category of items for which to shop. Yesterday's arrival had been a cushion that prevented the seatbelt from rubbing against Cali's port. The day before, a mug had arrived that read, Cancer Fucked with the Wrong Bitch.

Awesome.

Thanks for the coffee.

And the reminder that my wife has cancer.

Slurp.

I went online myself and was shocked by the huge market for cancer patients. It makes sense that part of the population has cancer on a rotating basis, and, therefore, people have profited from that. But there's something morbid about Shirley in Minnesota with a screen press in her basement, selling T-shirts on Etsy that read, Not Today, [insert type of cancer]!

Nonetheless, I, too, succumbed and ordered stickers for everyone in the family that read, In This Family, No One Fights Alone, over a green ribbon—the symbol for Lymphoma Awareness. I thought that would rally the troops.

On this day, for whatever reason, though, I did not ignore the doorbell's security camera alert, thinking perhaps some fool was trying to break into my house in broad daylight while everyone was home during COVID. On my phone screen, the video came up, and I saw my father-in-law dragging my empty garbage cans up from the end of the driveway. I masked up and went out through the garage.

"Hey, how's it going?" I asked. "Thanks for getting those."

I should have gotten those.

I try to act kind of cool and casual around Al. Like I've got everything under control. In reality, I actually never *do* have anything under control, have never *had* anything under control, and never *will* have anything under control.

"No problem," he said as he walked over to his car and reached inside, emerging with a large, brown paper bag. "I brought bagels. And a black-and-white cookie for my little Ella."

I was strangely unable to speak. My eyes became wet. Maybe allergies.

He looked at me standing there and ordered, "Come here," as he extended the arm not holding the bag.

He hugged me. A giant boulder hugged me.

We hugged longer than was customary in polite society, and I buried my tearstained face in the comfort of his puffy, blue down jacket. I gave him a one-handed shoulder pat to signal I was done, and he pulled back, looking away, also unable to speak. I'm not saying he was crying. Let's just leave it alone, unless you're looking for trouble.

"You need me. I'm here." He pointed his girthy digit at me.

It wasn't an offer; it was a command.

I went back in to work and called my colleague, Mitchell. As the phone rang, I reminisced.

★★★

It was 1999, and Mitchell and I had just finished our business dinner in a little cottage on the outskirts of Antwerp. The week had started off terribly, with our Belgian clients giving us a less-than-warm reception and making it clear they'd rather work with *ze Germans*. But by the time Mitchell and I had jumped through all their hoops and convinced the dry motherfuckers to have dinner with us that last night, we had figured out some of the cultural differences and were all laughing and joking around. These guys weren't bad, actually. We just had to warm up to each other.

We shook hands with Nergen, Flurgen, and Jurgen and bid them *goedenacht*. It was 10 p.m. on Thursday night, and we were *finally done*.

We weren't scheduled to fly back to the states until Sunday. This was back when you'd get a much cheaper flight if you stayed over the weekend—enough to justify the extra room and board—so we had time to kill, and I was looking forward to it. I didn't have kids then and while I missed Cali, just chilling at the weird hotel with Mitchell sounded fine to me after the week we'd had.

We walked to our rental car, and I felt an incredible sense of relief. The meetings were over, our mission was accomplished, and most importantly, we were finished. Overseas business trips can take a lot out of you. As we stood outside the car, about to get in, Mitchell paused by the driver's side and looked at me over the roof of the dark-green Renault. "Want to drive to Paris?"

What I wanted was to go to sleep for three days and then sleep on the plane and then sleep some more when I got home. "I guess?" I ventured.

I didn't know exactly where in the world we were, nor where Paris was in relation. This was only my second or third trip to Belgium, although I would wind up going there many times during the next several years as we grew our business.

So we drove to Paris.

It was three and a half hours, but Mitchell kept me entertained the whole time. We reminisced about our awkward meetings, listened to music, and laughed.

"That guy fully picked his nose and wiped it on his shirt while he was talking. Is that a Belgian thing, or is he just disgusting?"

"I'm gonna learn Flemish so that next time, I can understand what they're saying about us behind our backs."

This was pre-smartphone, so I didn't have some navigation system running. Maybe we had one of those early rental navigation units, but I'm not sure if that was a thing yet either. A MapQuest printout would have been handy, but this was a spontaneous trip, and we had nothing. Mitchell said not to worry. He had spent plenty of time in Paris and knew exactly where we were going.

As we approached, though, Mitchell seemed less and less sure about where we were. We were definitely in the vicinity of Paris, but we seemed to be going in circles, weaving through the outskirts and through some surprisingly heavy traffic for that time of night.

I thought about the scene from *National Lampoon's European Vacation* when the Griswolds were endlessly stuck in a traffic circle. "Hey, look, kids, there's Big Ben, and there's Parliament."

"What's that sign say?" Mitchell asked with urgency as he concentrated on grinding the stick shift and navigating merging lanes of traffic without killing us.

I'd taken Spanish in high school. French always seemed to have too many extra letters and accents and silent letters. And I felt silly pronouncing French words properly.

I looked at the sign. It said *Rue de la Paix.*

"I don't know," I told him. "Rue de la Paikes? Pay? Pah? How do you pronounce P-A-I-X?"

By the time I said that, we were two blocks past the turn anyway. We were lost.

After an extra forty-five minutes of driving in circles, cutting off angry French drivers, and laughing our asses off, we finally screeched to a stop in front of the *Hôtel Américain.* We checked in and headed up to our rooms. Sweet Lord, I was going to sleep well.

I put my key in the door and looked over at Mitchell, who was one door down doing the same. I opened my mouth to bid him *adieu,* figuring we'd do some light touristy things the next day, when he said, "Meet me in the lobby in twenty minutes."

It was 1 a.m.

A half hour later, I was following Mitchell down a cobblestone street and then into a dark alley. He was on autopilot now, having gotten his bearings, and knew exactly where we were headed. I wouldn't have noticed the door in the alley if he hadn't stopped abruptly. No one was around. There were no markings on the door. No signs overhead.

We crossed the threshold and walked down a long, dark staircase. I could hear the bass pumping.

Oontz, oontz, oontz, oontz.

It grew louder as we descended, and now I could *feel* the bass pumping. It filled my head and thumped in my chest.

OONTZ, OONTZ, OONTZ, OONTZ.

Neon lights and lasers flashed across my vision as we entered the somehow incredibly crowded nightclub. I grew slightly nervous. This wasn't my scene. Mitchell looked back at me, laughing and waving me toward the bar. By the time I caught up, he was already lining up shots and inviting people into our circle of trust.

That night was a booming, neon, boozy blur. We laughed, drank, danced, and maybe (innocently) flirted with some Parisian women as we bar-hopped across Paris. I felt incredibly alive and awake after a brutal week. Mitchell and I had trudged through some shit together in those meetings, but that night we celebrated making it through. It was better than sleeping, that was for sure.

In a taxi back to the hotel around 7 a.m., through the ringing in my ears, I heard "Hotel California" come on the radio. It felt like a sweet taste of the good old US of A after all the German techno still pounding in my head. Mitchell and I started singing at the top of our lungs.

Three lines into the song, the French driver leaned forward, and without saying a word, clicked the radio off. Mitchell and I looked at each other in the uncomfortable silence, our eyes wide and our mouths open in surprise. Then Mitchell continued singing even louder.

I joined him. It isn't a short song, and we knew every word. The driver was not amused.

Fucking Americans ....

Mitchell was giggling.

We had a wild night thanks to that maniac.

Oh, right. I should have mentioned that Mitchell is my boss and the owner of the company where I've worked for over twenty-six years.

That night was over twenty years ago. Before and since then, Mitchell and I have slain many dragons together and shared many adventures like that night in Paris.

Although he could wake up tomorrow and decide to fire me, I try not to think about that. He's like a brother to me. A wealthy brother who can end my career on a whim, but a brother nonetheless.

★★★

So now, I was returning Mitchell's call. He had been doing some thinking. He had a family doctor who was well-connected at Memorial Sloan Kettering in the city, which, if you don't already know, is the *crème de la crème* for cancer treatment.

Hey, *crème de la crème*. Maybe I do speak *Franchez*.

Anyway, all I had to do was say the word, and Mitchell would make the connections and get Cali in to see the top lymphatic specialist, ironically named Dr. Limpf Node.

That's not really his name. I don't remember his name.

Truth be told, I had actually been thinking about us getting a second opinion. It certainly seemed like a thing people do. In fact, almost anyone who knew about Cali eventually asked if we were either getting a second opinion or going to Memorial Sloan Kettering (MSK). Apparently, that was what you did if you got cancer. You got a second opinion, and you went to MSK.

I couldn't understand what good it would do. Would they say Cali's diagnosis was wrong, and she *didn't* have cancer? Would they propose some radical homeopathic treatment that could only be performed in the rain forest of the Yucatán?

Yes, lady, lie in this mud bath and eat crickets while we rearrange your chakras.

Also, Cali was supposed to be starting her treatment that Monday. It was Friday, March 5. The sooner we got started, the sooner we would be finished. I didn't want to delay things at least two weeks while we considered other doctors and treatments.

Most importantly, Cali loved her current team. She had already gotten to know and trust them during her search for answers and the iron infusions. And as much as I tease Dr. Gingerpubes, he was with Cali every step of the way so far and was clearly an excellent doctor.

On top of everything, my mother-in-law *hates* Memorial Sloan Kettering. She knew three people who'd died under their care. It didn't matter if they'd been beyond help or what the details had been, Arlene didn't trust MSK anymore as a result. So, it was going to be a huge pain in the ass if I wanted to convince Cali to change up the entire plan.

I told Mitchell to go ahead and make the phone call.

Two hours later, my phone rang. It was Dr. Node from MSK. He sounded important, old, and busy. He sounded like he had a thick beard and thicker glasses. He told me he understood I had some close friends at MSK, and he was happy to clear time in his schedule to see Cali.

Not exactly accurate, but I didn't correct him.

"When would you like to come in?" he asked matter-of-factly.

I hemmed and hawed, saying I'd like to explain what was going on with Cali first. He asked me to break down the situation for him, which I did. How it had started, how it was eventually diagnosed, and when the R-CHOP treatment was prescribed.

Dr. Node agreed that R-CHOP was the way to go nowadays. Ever since they added the R to CHOP, it had become a completely different success rate. He actually said that. CHOP? Not so much. R-CHOP? Much better.

But did I happen to know the precise histologic subtype? And if it was nodal or extra-nodal? *Um, what?*

He'd lost me, which I had expected but was hoping wouldn't happen. So, I asked him something that felt stupid at the time, but maybe it was just straight to the point. "Is that something that any normal doctor would ask?"

He was quiet again, not sure what to make of me.

I cut the bullshit. "Dr. Node, I know that you are the best in the field, and that MSK is the best place to get care, and I really do appreciate you calling me. But my wife is very comfortable with her team and was planning to start treatment on Monday, so I am really just looking for some reassurance that we are following the right path. These questions you are asking, is this something Cali's doctor would consider as well?"

He was quiet for a second. Probably wondering what kind of a fool has a connection at MSK and doesn't take advantage of it.

He eventually said yes, this was the correct treatment, and any normal doctor would be asking and considering the same things. If we were comfortable with our current doctor, then we should continue with him by all means. There was no chance of the diagnosis being incorrect, nor was there any new or experimental wizardry on which we were missing out.

"I will notify Dr. So-and-So that I have called you. I will tell him that we spoke, and that you have declined to come in."

Favor fulfilled.

Still, I felt relieved about what he'd had to say. And technically, it *was* a second opinion.

CHAPTER 7
Tick-Fucking-Tock

I cracked three eggs into a bowl and mixed in a splash of half-and-half. That's the trick for fluffy omelets. I used to use milk, but all we had in the house lately was skim and almond milk and oat milk, and you may as well use water if you're going to use those. I took the leftover half of last night's French dip sandwich out of the fridge, and I peeled the cold steak off the garlic roll along with the now-hardened melted Swiss cheese. I threw that in a pan and sautéed it with onions over melted butter.

When it looked done, I put in some sliced cherry tomatoes and—screw it—poured the leftover au jus in there from the little cup. It sizzled, and I remembered to put on the vent fan just in time as the steam rose up. I had smoked out our kitchen one too many times and refused to get yelled at again. When some of that *au jus* cooked off, I whisked in the eggs, pulling in from around the edges with a spatula as it cooked.

You stay fluffy, San Diego, I thought, channeling the great Ron Burgundy from *Anchorman*.

After a while, I flipped the omelet, sprinkled on a little (read: a lot of) shredded mozzarella, and folded it over and onto my plate. Then I crisped the two sides of the leftover garlic bread from the former sandwich in the pan over some fresh butter and put them on the plate as well.

I have an imaginary restaurant in my head I will never open. I don't have too many details figured out except we will definitely serve breakfast and will definitely never open. I have a few concoctions that would be on the menu for sure, and this French dip omelet just might make the cut.

After breakfast, I cleaned the fish tank.

Then, I sorted through my desk drawers, cleaning out old papers and bills; I'd been meaning to do that for a while.

That got me to 11 a.m.

I was trying to fill time with various distractions because tomorrow was Cali's first day of chemo, and I was freaking the fuck out. Things had felt pretty real until now, but today they felt *really* real. Tomorrow, it would be official. Cali would go in there, and they'd plug into her port and expose her to all kinds of chemicals. There was no turning back after tomorrow. Not that we could turn back anyway.

For lunch, I took out the lobster roll kit from our friends Lee and Jessica via the Clam Shack in Maine. It was sent through Goldbelly, a website that ships famous foods from restaurants all over the country. Food was rolling in from everyone. I brushed melted butter onto the inside of the fresh rolls, grilling them to a golden brown. Then I put a smear of mayo on each roll top and stacked the lobster onto each bottom half. Finally, I squeezed some lemon, drizzled a little more melted butter on there, and dug in. Sweet Fancy Moses, they were delicious. I was going to become tremendous if I kept eating like this during Cali's treatment. Too late actually.

Now it was 1 p.m.

Tick-Fucking-Tock.

I thought about going for a walk with Cali. Cleaning the basement. Doing some work. Anything.

But suddenly, I could no longer function. I had no energy or desire to do anything. I didn't want to think, much less move. This would have been a good time to visit my local opium den. I could just lie there on a couch in the dark, listen to a mandolin, and puff from the hookah all day.

Is that a thing? Opium dens?

It had been a long day.

That night, Cali and I lay in bed, watching more *Deadwood*. When I get started with a show, I stick with it … and cowboys with tuberculosis are cool, I don't care what you say.

Anyway, the episode ended, and it was too late to start another. We had to be up early the next morning. Normally, if Cali is half asleep, I don't bother her when I turn in. I put on my incredibly sexy sleep apnea CPAP mask and strap in for my best impression of a chubby Darth Vader. Or if Cali is awake, we do a half-assed kiss goodnight—both of us too lazy to roll all the way over for a proper kiss, so we meet in the middle for a quick peck before we fall back to our sides, exhausted from the effort.

Who says romance is dead?

Tonight, however, I needed to connect with my wife. I sucked it up and rolled *all the way over* to her side. It was a big move. I placed my hand flat on her tiny, little chest. I still wasn't used to her bony frame. I felt her heart beating and looked into those green eyes.

"Get off me!" she whispered seductively.

Okay, it was more of an annoyed yell.

"Wait, wait. I just wanted to say that I love you. And you've got this, Cali. I'll be with you every step of the way."

Except I won't have the cancer and pain and chemotherapy and hair loss, and, oh, I won't be in the building either.

She must have smelled the onions from my steak omelet because her eyes teared up. "I'm so scared," she whispered.

I was scared too.

We tried to get some sleep.

★★★

I was carrying the pieces of a broken vase in my cupped hands, rushing to get it fixed. Then it morphed into a bashed-in old radio. Later, it changed into a large armful of loose mechanical parts I struggled to keep in my arms. No matter what form, it was clear the item was broken, and I was running to get it repaired. People I knew were offering to help, but I ran past them, knowing I had to do this myself. Much like when I grabbed baby Ella away from our nurse, Dorothy, I felt a sense of responsibility for correcting the situation personally.

I ran through my childhood home in Commack, Long Island. Right through the front door, down the hallway, past my parents who were standing there, and out the back door. I ran past Cali's parents as I sped through their old summer camp. Other family members and friends tried to stop me along the way in various familiar locales.

The broken item in my arms kept changing, but that did not seem unusual. The fact that it was getting larger with each transformation caused me concern. Eventually, I was no longer carrying an object in my arms as I ran. Instead, I was under it, like Atlas supporting the globe, but on my chest. I slowed to a labored walk. Ultimately, I fell to my knees and then lay flat on my back. What had now become a huge blob of amorphous energy was squashing me, compressing my chest. Crushing me. It began vibrating, about to explode.

I woke up to find Loki lying on my chest, purring away.

My dream was still with me. I could feel the panic.

It didn't take a rocket surgeon to figure that one out.

CHAPTER 8
No Turning Back

When my alarm went off at six forty-five, my body didn't want to move. My brain didn't want to think. I had been waking up at seven thirty this past year, which was much later than usual since I wasn't contending with a soul-crushing commute. There's always a bright side to a global pandemic, don't let them tell you otherwise. In recent days, though, I'd been driving Ella to school every other day to let Cali sleep. Six forty-five in the morning was the required wake-up time, and I was still adjusting. Good thing I hardly showered anymore.

It was March 8, 2021, and a touch warmer than usual that morning but still chilly. On the way to school, Ella seemed sad. I presumed it was about her mom, so I treated her to some of my best Dad Joke material. I'm sure her day was brightened.

Then I drove home to pick up Cali for her first treatment: the R in R-CHOP. This medication prepares the body for chemo. It is administered slowly to see how much the patient's body can handle, which determines how long the treatment lasts. We were warned of a reaction called *rigors* that can result from too much medication too soon. The name made me think of "rigor mortis," and I pictured Cali suddenly stiffening up and rising like a rigid but sexy little zombie. Or maybe it's called *rigors* because it is so *rigor*ous. Either way, breaking down the rigors to its Latin root wasn't making it sound any less terrible, so I stopped thinking about it.

I dropped Cali off outside the hospital. She was armed with her tablet, which I had spent all weekend loading up with movies, shows, and every streaming service known to man. She had a blanket and pillow and various other comforting items in a large beach tote. I pretended she was leaving on an international flight, but instead of serving mimosas, they plugged a drip into your chest hole and slowly poisoned you.

I drove home and received a text from Cali just as I pulled into the driveway. According to her blood test, her potassium something-something was low, so before they even started, they had to put her on a two-hour supplemental drip. Very important to level out the potassium.

I'm no Doogie Howser, but I wondered: *Couldn't they have just fed her a banana?*

Either way, it was shaping up to be a long day for Cali. She hadn't even started yet.

I entered our house and sat down in my office to get to work only to realize it was 10 a.m., and I was supposed to pick Ella up from school at 10:10 a.m.

What kind of insane school day was that? She was in school for less than three hours. What was the point?

I hopped back into the car and drove to the high school once again. I was sick of driving to this school. I was sick of driving back and forth to Northern Westchester Hospital. I was sick of driving, period. I was tempted to just swerve into a tree on the way there and call it a day. And this was *day one* of Cali's treatment—just to make it totally clear that I am a giant baby.

I told myself this misery I was experiencing was (a) nothing compared to what Cali was dealing with and (b) Cali's exact routine every day before we found out she was sick. Cali put more miles on her car each year in Somers than I did driving back and forth to the city each day. Cali drove to Target, to Stop & Shop, to drop the kids off, and to pick them up. She drove and drove and then drove some more. And when she got home, she remembered something she'd forgotten and headed back out again.

Or she was having an affair. Either way, it had been an impressive amount of driving.

I never really thought about it, but Cali had driven everywhere for everything and never complained once. I had done it for a few days and was ready to end it all in a fiery blast.

Thankfully, I managed to make it home in one piece with Ella, avoiding the surrounding Westchester reservoirs and other tempting hazards. I finally sat down to do some work and realized I had promised Ella we could practice driving.

More driving.

Ella was sixteen and had her learner's permit. She somehow had to log one hundred hours of driving before she could get her license. We had done probably forty-six minutes so far. And because we practiced so infrequently, each time we got in the car, it was like Ella's first time, and she'd forgotten half of what she learned.

We got in the car, and Ella adjusted her mirrors and seat, clearly killing time while she tried to remember how to start the car. I mentally planned out our route.

We live in The Woodlands. The neighborhood consists of 180 homes. When they were originally building, you could choose from three color selections and five models. The original landscaper was rumored to have stripped all the topsoil when they cleared out every tree and living thing in sight, which they were happy to sell back to me at a premium when we moved in. Either way, the landscaping was similar all around. The neighborhood isn't exactly cookie-cutter, but it's close.

Route 118 is the main road that runs north/south along the west side of The Woodlands. There are two entrances roughly three hundred yards apart from each other on the east side of 118. These two entrances lead to two roads that meet at the back corner of The Woodlands. Belmar, the first entrance, runs in a lazy semicircle for roughly a mile and a half. Toward the end, it intersects with the road from the second entrance, Pimlico. Pimlico runs straight for a mile until it meets back up with 118 at that second entrance. Our humble abode is past the intersection of Belmar and Pimlico, which is nice because there are only a handful of homes down that way until Belmar ends, so we don't get a lot of traffic. In between and off to the sides of Belmar and Pimlico are various connecting roads, and yes, to quote El Guapo from *Three Amigos*, I would say we have a "plethora" of *cul-de-sacs*, or "dead ends" as we used to call them when I was growing up.

More French lessons, but did you know the translation of *cul-de-sac* from French is literally "arse of the bag"? *Dead end* sounds better once you know that factoid.

Anyway, if you're thinking that all adds up to the perfect practice course for young Ella to test out her driving skills, you'd be wrong. With those 180 homes come 180 families. Those families mostly consist of two parents and two or three kids. Sure, some families are smaller, but some have Grandma and Grandpa living in the extra bedroom. So, let's just say the average household holds five people. That's nine hundred people wandering around.

Some families are young, and those kids like to play in the street, ride bikes, and I don't know, roll in the mud. Some families have older children, like mine, and those kids have cars. And it seems 179 of those 180 homes have dogs. And it seems 179 of those 180 homes, for some reason, do not use their garages or driveways for their intended purposes and, therefore, park on the street. And it seems 179 of those 180 homes have at least one semiprofessional track star or Olympic-hopeful power walker living there. And the roads are not, let's say, "wide" or "regulation." And many of the residents mistakenly believe that speed limits and stop signs are optional if they appear in your own neighborhood. The result is an insane obstacle course full of street-parked cars, narrow roads, joggers, walkers, carriages, dogs, pick-up basketball games, more dogs, and general chaos that drives me absolutely bonkers and makes my daughter terrified to drive.

Ah, the suburbs. So relaxing.

At some point during the drive, I took a break from pointing out life-threatening obstacles, and we started talking about college. Ella was a junior in high school at the time. At this point with our other two kids, we had already done some college visits and research. Due to COVID (again), schools weren't allowing in-person visits, which really should have made things easier since we could do limitless virtual visits from home, but we had been slacking. Every weekend, I'd tell Ella to grab me so we could sit and "do some college stuff." And every weekend passed, including this past one, and we neglected our duties. This being Monday, I reminded her we had forgotten once again.

"I know," she said. "We have to do some stuff this week. And the essay prompts came out for the common application, so we should look those over."

I thought for a moment then said, "Well, look on the bright side. You'll have something to write about now."

That afternoon, I headed back to the hospital. I parked in the roundabout under the No Parking No Standing Any Time sign, waiting for Cali to emerge. There was nowhere to pick up or drop off here due to all the makeshift tents and construction to accommodate COVID, so I figured I would just wait here and hope no one made me move. So far, it hadn't been an issue, but I couldn't believe this massive hospital relied on this tiny circular drive with nowhere to stop. Were we supposed to throw our loved ones out the window as we screeched through the curve? If it hadn't been for the CVS parking lot, I didn't know where I'd have gone during these appointments.

I could see the distant second entrance Cali used behind me in my right sideview mirror and was keeping my eye on it. I was ready to mask up and jump out of the car when she appeared. This was the time of year when the weather was completely unpredictable, and this afternoon, it had become too freaking cold for me to wait outside. However, I didn't know what kind of shape Cali would be in after her first day of treatment, and I wanted to at least run around to the other side of the car to open the door for her when she came out.

Man, she must have had some day, I thought.

I know she was terrified to go in there in the first place, not knowing what to expect. And she was alone. Then she endured hours of taking tests, waiting for results, getting supplements plugged into her port all before she even got to the main course: six hours of a drug that could cause the dreaded *rigors*. I looked at the clock on the dash. She had been there for more than eight hours. I bet she was exhausted.

I then wondered how quickly Cali would begin to feel the side effects. Dr. Clifford the Big Red Dog—sorry, ran out of redhead jokes—said days five to ten after treatment would be the toughest since that was when Cali's white blood cell count would be lowest.

But is it all relative? Will she feel sick tonight? Will her hair begin falling out right away?

Suddenly, it was difficult to breathe.

Goddamnit, it was official. There was no turning back.

When my wife comes through those doors, she'll have that poison in her.

This was all too real.

Then, Cali appeared in my sideview mirror—small and far away at the second entrance. According to my mirror, though, she was closer than she appeared, so I was on full alert. She emerged from the automatic doors and walked slowly and carefully down the ramp toward me. Another wave of nervous fear swept over me as I put on my mask, got out of the car, and began to make my way around the vehicle.

Instead of heading to the other side to open the door as I'd planned, I found myself running to her, tears welling up inside me.

Cali is only five foot one but normally gives a taller appearance. Today, she looked small.

Cali is always either tan from the sun or bronzed from, well, bronzer or spray-tanning. Today, her skin looked pale and gray.

Cali usually walks with a bit of a confident strut. Today, she seemed frail and moved slowly.

Maybe it was just cold and gray out, and she was tired. Half of it could have been my imagination, but my heart broke as I ran up to her and grabbed her arms, sobbing. Not the coolest move. "What did they do to you?"

"I'm fine," she said cheerfully.

"No, no, no," I moaned. "They broke you. They broke you, Cali. My wife, my wife. Why? *Why?*" I was losing my shit. This was not what I had planned.

I helped her into the car. When I came around and got in, I was still sobbing.

"Gregg, I am totally fine," Cali reassured me.

"Why, Cali? *Why?*" I could barely understand what the hell I was blubbering. "What did they to do you? They poisoned you. Oh my God! No, no, no."

I was yelling, sobbing, weeping, and blabbering all kinds of nonsense. For some reason, I started driving, even though I couldn't even see through the tears and my swollen eyes.

I'll spare you the rest. I somehow managed not to crash, and I haven't cried like that in a long time. Maybe ever, unless you count that time when I really wanted that bottle. But I was six months old then.

The cry was cathartic though.

I had been "brave" for Cali up until that moment. Then the dam broke, and the whole thing just hit me at once. The reality of it all—the crossing of some imaginary threshold—knowing poison was officially inside my wife, and there was no turning back.

The hopelessness.

The fear.

CHAPTER 9
The Rigors

Yesterday was the R, and today, March 9, Cali got the CHO. Tomorrow, she would take a P.

It reminded me of that old sign that said, "Welcome to our ool. Notice there is no P in it. Let's keep it that way."

I wanted to make a sign when this was all over: "Say hello to ali. Notice there is no big C in her anymore."

Hey, that's pretty good.

Turns out, Cali did have the pleasure of experiencing *the rigors* yesterday. They had gradually cranked up her dosage all morning, adjusting her to the medication but also determining the maximum she could handle. At one point, of course, just when the nurse took a bathroom break, Cali locked up. She said her teeth clenched together so hard and tight, she thought they were going to shatter. She began shivering uncontrollably. The nurses all jumped to her side, layering her with blankets and lowering the dosage until it passed.

Fun times.

After I dropped Cali off for her second treatment, I headed down to Westchester County Center to get my first dose of the Pfizer vaccine. I hadn't been vaccinated yet because I hadn't met the criteria. Naturally, when the first vaccine came out from Pfizer, it had been prioritized for the elderly, first-responders, and eventually teachers. The Moderna vaccine soon followed, but the qualifications were the same, and the supply was scarce.

Of course, I'd had opportunities to get it. My ice-fishing buddy, Fireman Mike, knew the guy working the vaccination site in Floral Park. His text at the time said that if I could get there within the hour, he would slip me in. Our other friend, who let's say is in the health-care industry, had extra doses. I'd just have to come around back.

There were other offers, but I'd passed on all of them. Not that I'm such a saint, but early on, when the vaccine was scarce, and COVID was really spreading, I couldn't help but think about whose dose I would be stealing. Someone who was on the front lines and really needed it, or someone who was ailing and would be in serious trouble if they got the big sick. Although, considering I lose my breath walking up my driveway after getting the mail, I was certain I'd be in big trouble, too, if I got it.

I still didn't take advantage though, even when Jacko, another one of my ice-fishing buddies, shared the news in our group text that now if your BMI was over thirty, you qualified. I did a quick mental inventory of the guys in the ice-fishing crew and was pretty sure he'd been talking to me.

So, I'm a big, lazy bastard, and as a result, I'm rewarded with the vaccine.

I had always hoped this giant belly would come in handy someday, but it didn't seem right. I even heard that smokers were qualifying in New Jersey. It was all ass-backward, but nothing surprised me anymore.

Anyway, things were loosening up a bit in the vaccination department. The Johnson & Johnson vaccine came out, and it was only a matter of time before there was a drive-through Olive Garden bottomless syringe vaccine or a Turbo Tax vaccine being dispensed at ATMs. More and more people we knew were vaccinated, and it seemed things had taken a turn. I no longer felt I'd be stealing someone else's dose. Between that and Cali being sick, I decided it was time to cash in the chubby chip.

It was a little embarrassing asking my doctor for a note saying I was technically obese and, therefore, needed the vaccine, but he didn't bust my chops too badly. Before I knew it, I was entering the vicinity of the

Westchester County Center. I had been here before. We had taken the kids to the Big City Circus to watch clowns abuse captive elephants years ago. Later, Alix and I had come here for the Lizard and Reptile Expo, which was a weird thing for the two of us to have done, now that I think about it. We bought a chameleon and a cage and lights and decorations and food and substrate. Hundreds of dollars. The chameleon, Doctor Pasquale Rosenpenis, passed away two months later. Rest in peace, Doctor.

The WCC looked a little different this time though. As I approached, the roads were narrowed by cones and emergency vehicles. Giant signs flashed Vaccination Parking. Uniformed police directed us. There was an armed military presence. Huge white tents were set up all around the main building. All I needed was an army chopper to fly low overhead and I'd be in the opening credits of a postapocalyptic thriller.

I parked and followed the clearly marked lines toward the building. I noticed they were geared up for a much larger crowd as I bypassed the empty and winding roped-off area set up for thousands of more people. I felt like a SuperPass customer at a major amusement park but entering a ride that was somehow even shittier than It's a [Tiny Planet,] After All.

It was around 11 a.m., and the weather had taken a positive turn. After a brutally cold and snowy few months, the temperature was up to a balmy fifty-six degrees. While driving farther and farther south to get here, there was less and less snow on the ground. By the time I reached White Plains, the only snow left was in a large, dirty pile plowed into the corner of the parking lot. The air was different too. It felt like spring.

I inhaled and couldn't help but to think metaphorically—you know, because I am so deep—that we had endured a cold winter, and now that Cali had started her treatment, we could begin the spring healing. Or maybe it's going to snow ten inches again tomorrow, and we're just entering the nightmare phase of Cali's long road.

I must admit, I was impressed with the situation there at the WCC. Since I didn't have much faith in the government at that point, I was amazed at what they had organized. There were clear lines to follow, armed personnel, and friendly, unarmed volunteers helping guide us every ten feet. It was overkill as each volunteer directed me to the next one who was waving frantically just a few feet away, but it was incredibly coordinated.

I wound my way through the guide ropes. Similar magical ropes had recently held off insurgents dressed as marauding Vikings in our nation's capital. I laughed to myself, remembering. Those fuckers had broken though barricades, knocked down cops, and smashed windows, but if you watch the videos, they all instinctively stayed within the velvet ropes while passing through the rotunda. Funny how the human mind works.

Anyway, I got my shot (didn't hurt) and my little sticker saying I'd been vaccinated (kept it). I was then corralled into the antechamber to wait the allotted fifteen minutes to make sure I didn't break out in hives or turn into a bat or something.

Cali texted me. I figured she'd be almost done with her treatment, so it was perfect timing.

Turns out her phosphorus was low again, so they had to transfuse her … or *in*fuse her … with phosphorus. Either way, they were just getting started. Next on the menu were two different anti-nausea meds, each of which would take forty-five minutes to administer. Then, there would be one hour of the chemo. In between, they had to clean out her blowhole (her port), of course. Bottom line, it was CVS-parking-lot time for me. I didn't want to go home in case anything went wrong and they needed me right away.

That afternoon, finally back home, I watched Cali carefully. I was fully prepared for her to start projectile vomiting like the girl from *The Exorcist* while her hair started falling out in patches until she looked like the Crypt-Keeper from *Tales of the Crypt*.

I told you, I've watched a lot of horror movies.

Surprisingly, Cali instead went for a walk with Ella, braving the mayhem out there in The Woodlands.

CHAPTER 10

A Giant Baby with a Hair-Trigger Temper

Cali's third day of treatment was supposed to be quick. In and out for a single shot. The P in R-CHOP. I planned on driving her there and waiting in my favorite parking lot. Today's medication had to be administered twenty-four hours after her last treatment, which had ended later than expected yesterday, so we weren't going in until the afternoon. I got some work done that morning, and it felt good to be productive and jump on a few things that had been hanging over my head.

Naturally, a few minutes into her supposed quick visit, Cali texted me, saying it was going to be a while. They wanted to do a blood test first, so it would take an hour to get the results before they could start … if the results were good.

I had a bunch of packages to drop for returns to Nordstrom, Amazon, lululemon, and Bloomingdale's. Cali's never-ending online shopping spree giveth and taketh away, but it always made me happy to have returns. There was a UPS place near the hospital, and as I drove, I passed a car wash.

A car wash … wow.

It had been an entire year since I had gotten a car wash. I remembered because it was early March 2020, just before everything shut down due to COVID. I also remembered because my car was filthy.

I walked into UPS, balancing an impossible stack of boxes, and my phone buzzed. It was Cali texting me that it was going to be a while longer for some reason or another. Weighing the timing, I decided I could squeeze in a car wash, so I drove over and got in line.

As I waited three cars back, my phone rang. It was the head of our company's printing department, Eric Simon. He was on press in our Virginia factory with a production run for one of my accounts and noticed something strange. There were tiny little specks all over the front panel of a folding carton we'd been producing for an important project. The specks were in the customer's original art, so we hadn't questioned it up front, but on press it looked like a mistake. Eric was texting me photos but needed an answer within a half hour as to whether or not they should fix it; otherwise, they couldn't hold the press any longer and would have to pull the job.

I've always wanted to yell, "Stop the presses!" However, this would impact the critical delivery date, which was rapidly approaching, just like eighty other critical delivery dates we were juggling.

As I spoke to Eric, I crept forward to the next spot in the line of cars, which I now regretted entering.

Cali called immediately after I'd hung up to say they got the blood test results, and her numbers were off, so they needed to give her a supplement before administering the medication. I cringed.

The line shifted forward, putting me at the front now. I got out of the car, pulling on my mask, my cell phone precariously balanced between my ear and shoulder. Cali was saying the supplement would take a while. I told the guy working there I wanted the executive, undercarriage, wheel-brightening, rust-protection bullshit option, knowing they would just run it through the same conveyor of filthy brushes no matter what I chose. I then attempted to pay, text the photos of the press sheet, text the kids with an update, and explain the situation to my customer. All this with my face mask muffling my voice and causing me to sweat, and while trying not to touch any surface covered with a deadly virus. In addition, that new, constant buzzing in the back of my head was running on repeat: *mywifeissick, mywifeissick, mywifeissick, mywifeissick.*

I was frazzled.

I continued juggling as I watched my car move slowly through the wash. After they finished hand-drying it, I tipped the guys and hopped in the car. As I was headed back to the hospital, I played a fun game of noticing every streak and missed spot on the car, getting more and more angry for no good reason. I was pissed off, stressed, tired, and feeling sorry for myself.

I'm telling you all this in my defense, ladies and gentlemen of the jury. I'm not proud of this next part.

I picked Cali up, and she immediately began listing everything we had to do in the next few weeks. She was on high-energy for whatever reason, maybe because she was full of more steroids than Arnold Schwarzenegger in the eighties, but all I wanted to do was get home and collapse. I have a very low bandwidth for activity in general, and today had been a lot.

And yes, I am aware I am not the one with cancer, okay? But it's all relative, and I was shot. I would also like to submit into evidence, Your Honor, that I suffer from ADD, and my meds tend to fade in the afternoon, along with my attention span and patience.

"Oh!" Cali remembered, after bombarding me with the next few days' appointments, activities, prescriptions to be filled, and general errands to be done. "Can you just swing by the post office on the way home? I need to mail something."

I was on the ropes after being pummeled by the heavyweight champion of listing shit to do, Iron Cali GOOOOOOLDMAN. I was indeed ready to rumble. "No," I said flatly. "I'm done."

"Come on, I just need to get this done."

"We can do it tomorrow."

"Fine," she said.

Something about her tone led me to believe it was not fine. "Why do you say *fine* that way? What the fuck, Cali? I haven't done enough today?"

"Oh, *I'm sorry*. Did *you* go through chemo this week? You must be *exhausted*."

"*No*, Cali!" I heard myself yelling. "But I'm allowed to get tired! I am stressed the fuck out, and I am not going to the fucking post office!"

Cali looked at me for a second. "Oh, sorry I have *cancer*, and it is *so inconvenient* for you!" She was half-yelling and half-crying, tears running down her cheeks.

We drove in silence for a while.

Shit.

I immediately felt awful. I'd known I was bound to pull this shit at some point because I am a giant baby with a hair-trigger temper. It was just a lot sooner than I'd expected, so that was something to be proud of. "I'm really sorry," I said eventually.

"It's okay."

It wasn't okay.

Goddamnit.

I screwed up. I have no self-control.

We were quiet for a while longer, each lost in our own miserable thoughts. If I'd had a time machine at that moment, I wouldn't have gone back to 1986, like I'd always planned (to stop myself from wearing parachute pants). I would've gone back ten minutes and made a right turn to the post office.

We eventually pulled into our driveway.

Cali said, "This whole thing is weird. It's okay. Really. We are both stressed out, and it is going to happen again, I'm sure."

I breathed out a sigh of relief. "Thank you. I love you. Thank you for forgiving me."

What a saint. She was right though. It would happen again.

CHAPTER 11
The Asshole Theory

Cali didn't have any doctor appointments that Thursday, and I actually got a lot done at work, which felt great. I had a few Zoom meetings—they became a big thing during the pandemic—one of which was particularly significant.

I had been hesitant to tell any of my customers what was going on because, in my own experience, I never wanted to hear about other peoples' personal problems. It was a downer, and I preferred to skip all that and get work done. So I suppose I'd been projecting a little when I figured no one would want to hear what was going on with us.

That afternoon, however, I was forced to tell a customer—mostly because I had rescheduled the same meeting with her three times now, and I could tell she was starting to get irritated. We were on a Zoom conference call but with no video, and I was glad for that because, once again, my allergies started acting up as soon as I started explaining. I had only begun working with this woman a year ago, but she was so sweet and sounded so genuinely concerned about Cali and our family, that at first I thought she was full of shit. But no one can keep it going that long, and I could tell she really was dismayed.

My theory that most people are assholes was really being tested.

After many questions about Cali, she eventually asked me, "What are you doing to take care of *yourself?*"

I was silent. That was a stumper.

I made something up, but there was no real answer. Taking care of myself seemed like the most selfish thing to think about right now. I had to be *all in* for Cali. I had to sacrifice, suffer, and be completely miserable. When this was all over, I wouldn't have done my job unless I came out of it gray-haired with giant bags under my eyes, having aged twenty years and gained twenty pounds. Right? Isn't that how it works?

That evening, I was lying on the couch for some much-needed downtime when I got a text from Michael Y. He and Brenda were out walking, and they had "a little something" to drop off for Cali. Should they leave it, or was I around?

I typed that they should leave it but didn't hit send. I just stared at my phone for a good minute. I was thinking about these two people, Brenda and Michael, who genuinely loved Cali and cared enough to pick up a gift. These two had never given up on us, no matter how many times we flaked or canceled on them, and they were currently walking toward my house. It was pretty shitty that I was just going to tell them to leave it on the doorstep when all I was doing was scrolling through Instagram. That couldn't be how most humans acted, right? I then decided to join the human race one step at a time.

I deleted the unsent text and wrote that I'd be right out.

It was sunny but still a bit chilly when I saw Brenda and Michael walking up the front lawn with their little cockapoo, Jet. Jet is cute and soft and small, but he's also a little all over the place. He's just really excited to be around and see and smell stuff, so as a result, it's hard to connect with him. He loves to play fetch with a tennis ball, but he doesn't know when to stop.

I'm a renowned dog- and kid-whisperer, and although Jet and I haven't totally bonded after all these years, we're cool. Also, there are sixty dogs the exact breed, size, and color as Jet in our neighborhood, so I may be confusing him with one of them.

Anyway, Jet was cool today. Maybe he was tired from walking so much already, but he took a few scratches behind the ear and let it go, heading over to sniff a bush. I sat on the front steps, and Cali came out too, while Brenda and Michael stood at a careful six-foot distance from us on the walkway. Cali and I wore masks, but I told our visitors they could take theirs off. We were outside, socially distanced, and it seemed like overkill for everyone to have masks as long as Cali and I were packing.

Turns out, the gift they had was from Cali's whole crew of ladies. I don't remember what it was exactly, but it made Cali cry and was really thoughtful and nice with a beautiful card and everything. Then we spent the next forty-five minutes just talking with our visitors. I stayed focused, forcing my mind to come back if it began to wander. I don't have to tell you what it's like to space out, but ADD adds a new level of difficulty. The way my mind works when the meds have worn off is a bit like this:

Brenda: "Oh, you had your kitchen cabinets painted recently, right? How'd they come out?"

Cali: "Great! We were so worried at first ..."

Me: *Oh, yeah, that's right. Brenda went to Wisconsin, and she's only, like, two years younger than me. I wonder if she knew Amy What's-her-face? Man, that was fun when we used to road-trip to Madison, Wisconsin, from Michigan State. I think that was the first time I took mushrooms. Yeah, it definitely was. Oh man, I bugged out that first time. I remember we all walked into an arcade at one point while wandering the campus and town. I hadn't seen an arcade game since I was in sixth grade at the roller rink, playing* Zaxxon. *And the only video game I ever played in college was* Sega Hockey. *I was suddenly surrounded by games I had never seen, like* Mortal Kombat, *and the ultra-violence was really disturbing me. A dark-red curtain lowered in front of my eyes, and I began freaking out. But then, I remembered something one of the guys told me earlier as we ate mushroom sandwiches on white bread in the hotel room. I was in total control of my experience. So, I simply walked out of the arcade, taking a giant deep breath of clean, fresh air, and the dark-red curtain immediately lifted. And guess what? Half the other guys I was tripping with felt the same way and were all out there gasping for air too. We all looked at each other and laughed, feeling the crazy serendipity—*

"Right, Gregg?" Cali would be staring at me like, *Oh boy, we lost him again.*

So, I made a real effort to not do that this time around and managed to hang in there during the conversation. And I kept reminding myself, *These people care about us. These are good people. People connect with other people. That's what they do.*

I allowed myself to open up. I didn't even get defensive when Michael asked why the siding was so dented around my garage. It was from five years ago, when we'd had a basketball hoop in the driveway, and the kids smashed the shit out of the house with every missed shot or airball.

Okay, maybe that was me.

"Yeah, never got around to fixing that," I said.

He looked at me like he couldn't fathom how I could let something like that go unattended for so long.

I shrugged. *Whatever, man.*

This was cool. Hanging out, feeling the love, not feeling defensive or attacked or insecure or superior or overthinking things at all. I could get into this. It was nice. I just had to put myself out there.

One more thing about that visit.

When Cali first told her friends about her diagnosis, they had immediately offered to put together a Meal Train. I did not know what a Meal Train was, but Cali immediately told them they were not to put one together under any circumstances.

When I'd asked about it later, she explained, "They all sign up for slots on the calendar to make or send us dinner."

I'd thought about that. Cali was not going to be in any shape to cook. I love cooking, but my specialty is mostly over-grilling burgers to a crisp. And it stresses Cali out when I cook because I make such a mess. However, I had imagined I would cook on occasion during this whole thing. I figured that me cooking, coupled with ordering in a few nights, would do the trick and take any pressure off Cali, especially since it was just the three of us while the other two kids were still at school.

But this Meal Train deal meant that on certain nights, someone would just *drop off* a home-cooked meal. Or have something delivered. Not that I was overly concerned about it financially, but still, a *free* meal with no prep or clean up? No deciding or ordering? Zero hassle aside from maybe returning a container or two? It sounded incredibly helpful and convenient.

Why on Earth would we say no to that?

"I don't need someone else's food in my house," Cali explained.

Sorry, what?

That made zero sense. But she felt so strongly about it, and gave no further explanation, so I applied my new Zen-like attitude and agreed. No Meal Train.

That had been two weeks ago though, and maybe I didn't let it go entirely.

Every night at dinner, I'd say something like, "Wouldn't it have been nice if this was a Meal Train night? No hassle, blah blah blah."

And Cali would say something like, "Yuck."

Brenda had been the ringleader of the Meal Train proposal, so when Cali went inside for a minute, Brenda asked me about it again. Luckily, Brenda knew Cali well enough to accept the *yuck* without further explanation. I told Brenda to convince her though. When Cali came back out, Brenda bombarded her, and Cali finally acquiesced.

Yes!

We would soon be awash in the fruit of others' labor. Delicious home-cooked meals served up to our front doorstep in steaming, hot trays. Exotic dishes that were the specialties of other homes and unique to ours. A vacation for our taste buds, if you will. This may be the closest I ever got to swinging, and I was excited.

I love food.

Important note: That night, Cali said she could no longer feel some of the lymph nodes that had been poking out of her skin a few days ago. That was encouraging to hear.

CHAPTER 12

Ice Cream: Works Every Time

On Friday, we were looking forward to a second day of zero appointments, but Dr. Hopewell's office called to say he wanted Cali to come in for some blood work to check her levels. I pictured the doc in overalls with a long dipstick and a dirty rag, saying, "Top her off a quart of type O with extra magnesium."

Her appointment was for 10 a.m., and I figured I'd hang around since they said it would be quick.

Sucker.

I could do the drive in my sleep at this point, which I may have actually done that morning, now that I think about it. The drive was beginning to feel shorter each time, which was good. We left at 9:25 a.m. and arrived at the front door of the hospital at 9:55 a.m., and then Cali went in. I drove across the street and assumed the position. I responded to some work emails, figuring I'd be out of there in thirty minutes.

Twenty minutes in, Cali texted that they were going to need an hour to get the blood test results, so I should hang tight. After 11 a.m., Cali texted that her phosphorus was low and would take an hour. They were waiting for the rest of the lab results.

Phosphorus? Before all this started, I hadn't even known that was in us. I thought phosphorus was in road flares. I imagined the nurse approaching Cali with a red stick. There would be a loud *fwoosh* sound, and sparks would shower everywhere. "This will sting a little."

Aside from road flares, I pictured glowing algae in a cove somewhere in St. Lucia.

See how smart I am? I would have been a great marine biologist.

Ha, marine biologist.

That reminds me of when, early in our relationship, before we had kids, Cali and I took a trip to San Francisco. After a few days in the city, we headed south in a rental car to Monterey. We stayed at a bed-and-breakfast on the water called the Seven Gables Inn. It was fancy for us, and we were splurging.

I'd never do this today, but one thing about this place was that breakfast was kind of a communal thing. It was served at a specific time, so we found ourselves sitting around a large rectangular dining table with several other couples, eating dandelion pancakes or some other locally sourced concoction from the proprietor's garden. We made idle chitchat with our fellow travelers, and when they asked what our plans were for the day, we explained we were headed to the Monterey Bay Aquarium. Back then, Cali and I did a lot of traditional date things, like walking around malls and towns or going to movies, mini-golf, and bowling. We didn't care what we did as long as we were together. We always visited the local aquarium if they had one.

"I hear the Monterey Bay Aquarium is larger than the one in Boston," I informed Cali in front of our new friends.

"I hope they have baby belugas, like the one in Coney Island," Cali said to me.

"Yeah, or those hands-on displays, like in Mystic Seaport."

We continued to reminisce about our disproportionate history with aquarium visits, naming several others in the process.

One woman asked us excitedly, "Oh, are you marine biologists?"

Cali and I looked at each other. "Yes. Yes, we are."

We kept them going for a while. It was fun.

Phosphorus, right. Focus.

Another twenty minutes later, Cali texted again and said her potassium and other numbers were also low, so it would be another hour to drip in supplements. I considered sitting around and waiting. If I drove home, I would have to turn around and come back by the time I got there.

Ten minutes went by, and Cali texted again.
More like 3 hours

I started the car, thinking I'd run some errands.
Bzzzt.
More like 4 hours

Poor girl.

I drove home. I ate lunch. Did a little work. Got in the car and went back.

Cali got in the car and immediately started crying. "I'm so exhausted!" she sobbed. "I wasn't expecting to have anything today. I just want this to be over."

I gave her my line that this was a marathon, not a sprint. It's a decent metaphor I use when something sucks and is going to take a while. Coming from me, it means almost nothing since I've never run a marathon nor a sprint at any point in my life and never will.

Cali stared at me blankly.

I changed tactics, trying to get her back to focusing on what was right in front of her, one step at a time. That always helped me if I was facing a daunting task that seemed overwhelming. One baby step at a time. But that was usually a big project at work, not a battle for my life against cancer.

Everything I said felt empty as we continued to drive. She was so tired and frustrated.

I suddenly hit the brakes and made a hard right into a strip mall parking lot. "What do you want from Carvel?" I asked.

Cali sniffled, looking up at the Carvel sign. She wanted a soft-serve vanilla-and-chocolate swirl on a wafer cone, please. I went in and ordered, abstaining from getting anything for myself, believe it or not. It took an equal measure of willpower to avoid licking hers on the walk back to the car. I could have easily claimed it was melting, and

I had to stop the dripping. Anyone would believe that. I made it back to the car without caving, handed the cone over to Cali, and she ate it up like a little kid. She was happy for a few moments.

Ice cream. Works every time.

Our reprieve from reality was short-lived though, because as I pulled out of the lot, Cali's phone rang. It was the doctor's office. They called in a prescription to supplement some of her missing road flare juice (phosphorus), but it was only available at a pharmacy back in Bedford. It was nearby, but we had to turn around just when we thought we were done.

I pictured Al Pacino in *The Godfather Part III*. "Just when I thought I was out, they pull me back in!"

That movie sucks. I'm embarrassed I just quoted it. I apologize.

Leaving Cali in the car, I entered the pharmacy and joined the line at the back. It was five people deep. The woman working the counter seemed bored. She kept pulling her mask down and sipping a giant iced coffee. You'd think the coffee would have given her some energy, but maybe it hadn't kicked in yet. Maybe it was decaf. I cringed each time her mask came down, imagining the escaping particles floating toward my airholes.

The pharmacy had put little red circles on the floor. Each had a message asking us to please stay six feet apart. No one paid them any heed, which stressed me out. The woman in front of me was in shorts. She wore bright-red socks and clashing pink-and-purple tie-dyed Crocs. I was mesmerized. A young fellow who was also ahead of me was wearing work boots and a dark-blue jumper. He was covered head to toe in dried mud, and there was a Pig-Pen–like dust cloud hovering around him. I studied each person, noticing the face coverings were being worn like life preservers at summer camp. Just enough to be following the rules, but too loose to actually do anything.

I held my breath but only lasted fifteen seconds before I had to breathe again. I would make a terrible Navy SEAL. I gave up and began breathing normally, imagining COVID and dust flowing around my mask and into my lungs. Christ, I hated being in public, then and now.

When I finally made it to the front of the line, the bored coffee-sipper informed me they had just received our prescription. Which was bullshit since I knew the doctor's office had called it in at least forty-five minutes ago. She would expedite it for me, but I'd have to wait twenty minutes or so. I texted Cali the deal and then wandered around the pharmacy, carefully avoiding people like I was clearing a minefield in the Quang Tri Province.

Sometimes I feel like a timetraveler, or someone who has just emerged from a five-year coma. It was becoming increasingly apparent that Cali does everything for us. Conversely, I do nothing that isn't work-related. As a result, I hadn't been in a pharmacy for quite some time. I looked around, impressed with the revised layout and wide variety of products available to me here. This was less like a pharmacy and more like a mini-Walmart. If you needed a pool toy in early March, they had a section for that. If you needed pet supplies, they had a section for that. They even had a beer section with a few decent choices, which was surprising and kept me busy for a few minutes.

Just browsing. Keep moving, tubby.

What else had changed out here in the world during my period of laziness and subsequent quarantine?

By the time they called my name at the back desk, I had accumulated an armful of useless items. And Cali kept texting me requests from the car.

Get allergy meds, she remembered. Get me lip balm.

I paid and walked out, heading to the car where Cali was waiting. She was on the phone, I assumed with her mom. She was crying again. My sad Cali was five cars down. As I walked through the parking lot, I pulled my shirt up to my chest, exposing my giant belly. I rubbed it, like I had just eaten a delicious meal, swaying my hips, crossing my eyes, and licking my lips. I walked past a guy sitting in his pickup truck, and he stared at me.

Cali laughed though, so it was worth it.

CHAPTER 13
The In-Between

Since Cali did not have any appointments that lovely St. Patrick's Day, I scheduled a few early morning Zoom calls with customers to catch up on projects. My meetings began at 8:30 a.m. and went back-to-back for a few hours. The rapid-fire meetings were draining, but it was also exhilarating to speak to people and catch up with them personally and professionally. I was fired up to crank out some more work and then transition into a relaxing evening, my first day in a while without being in the car at all.

During my meetings, however, Cali popped into my office to tell me they had called in another phosphorus supplement prescription for her. The problem was it could only be filled at the CVS back near the hospital. I guess I was driving after all. And, driving back to the vicinity of the hospital even though we had no appointments. That was like driving into the city on a weekend back when I used to commute into midtown every weekday.

I finished my meetings and drove toward the CVS, figuring I'd at least be able to hit their drive-through since the prescription was already called in. On the way, Cali texted me, asking for Skippy Smooth Peanut Butter, which was totally random. Scratch that drive-through idea. I would have to go in and brave the masses once more.

Maybe bored iced coffee lady would be working. Or I'd see tie-dyed Croc woman. That would be exciting.

Anyway, they didn't have Skippy Smooth Peanut Butter at the CVS. They only had Skippy Super Chunk Extra Crunchy, but I had danced with this devil before.

Only get what was specifically requested. No substitutes will be accepted.

I was going to have to hit the grocery store.

Have you ever gone grocery shopping? I have, once or twice. It stresses me the fuck out. It normally goes like this:

I drive into the lot and search for a spot. People are walking right down the middle, completely unaware there may be cars driving through a parking lot. In fact, I've never driven through a parking lot when someone wasn't walking right down the middle of the lane, moseying along like they're in a field somewhere. I slowly roll the car up behind them, hoping the noise of the engine and the tires on gravel are enough to signal to them that I am present. But, no, they do not take notice. I consider honking, but I am not skilled enough on the horn to give a polite *tap* honk, and I fear I may accidently blast a louder and longer *GETTHEFUCKOUTOFTHEWAY* honk, so I hold off. I just roll along at less than one mile per hour behind the oblivious asshole meandering along at a snail's pace until they either get to their vehicle or somehow notice that, yes, there are other people on this planet, and one of them is about to run them over.

Incidentally, when *I'm* walking through a parking lot, I have two goals: (1) get to my car and (2) do not get hit by other cars. I pay attention.

I eventually manage to park without running anyone over, usually next to someone parked at a full 45-degree angle, and I must resist the urge to rip their side-view mirror off. I walk up to the storefront to select my shopping cart. The first two carts are always stuck together. The metals have intertwined somehow, bending the laws of physics, and no amount of human strength will pull them apart. I try anyway and fail.

The next cart comes free, but the front wheel is wobbly. I think I can deal with it, but after a few steps, it is pulling hard to the left, and

I don't have the muscle power to control that beast for the next hour. I return it. The next cart has a coupon circular in the basket, and that just bothers me. I'm not taking the paper out because the person before me was too lazy. Fuck them, I'm not cleaning up for someone else. I'm also not walking around with those coupons staring at me the whole time, serving as a constant reminder of the failures of the human race. I finally find a proper cart and mosey inside.

This is where I get *really* stressed out.

Imagine a movie scene where they mount the fish-eye camera on a dolly right in the main character's face. As they roll through the aisles, all you can see is a close-up of their distorted face, a drop of sweat easing down the forehead, eyes nervously twitching from left to right, and a little bit of the grocery store behind them. That's how I feel when I'm in the grocery store.

I have a list. It is in aisle order because my wife made the list, and she is insane and has this place memorized. I pray that nothing on the list has to go into one of those thin, plastic produce bags because I cannot pull them off the roll. I don't know where they start and where they end. If I do get a bag separated, I do not know which end opens. If I do get the bag open and put the product inside, I do not know how to close it. I also do not know how to handle this unlabeled item with no UPC at self-checkout. So, I try to stick to the prepackaged goods. I once needed a lemon for a recipe but purchased two dozen instead because they came in a labeled bag, which was easier to scan.

The list is written neatly. If there were a font called Kindergarten Teacher, it would be a replica of Cali's handwriting. Cali was a kindergarten teacher for ten years, by the way, so it makes sense.

It is not a TOOMAH!

Sorry, I am compelled to yell that in Arnold's accent if I hear the word "kindergarten."

Anyway, back to the list. If Cali makes a mistake while writing the grocery list, she does not cross or scribble it out, like you or I might. She rewrites the *entire list*.

Although neat, I pray nothing on the list is out of order. Cali's list is normally incredibly accurate. Start at the entrance and begin with veggies and fruit in the produce area. Easy. Wrap around to the far end for a little seafood and meat before turning back and hitting the juices and cereals. Cool. Just before the pharmacy and its adjoining cold remedies section, there is the seasonal aisle. You may find Valentine's Day or Halloween candy there. You may see Christmas decorations. Or, this time of year, various leprechaun or Easter bunny supplies. At just the right time of year, I am most happy to see tiki torches, coolers, and outdoor BBQ supplies, reminding me that warmer days are ahead. After that, I can work my way toward the home stretch where we have the frozen foods section and then the dairy aisle.

Occasionally, there's a random item on that shopping list that isn't where Cali thought it should be. That's when I must enter the *in-between*. Breadcrumbs? You're fucked. Pancake batter? Time to go home. When I enter the in-between, it is a showdown between my pride and the clock. Do I admit defeat and call Cali to ask where something is? Do I ask an employee for help? Or do I slowly lose my mind, wandering the in-between, perhaps never to return?

Another caveat I have when grocery shopping is that I will not, under any circumstances, go to the deli counter. That's a shit show, and I'd rather eat prepackaged deli meats.

All that aside, my biggest problem is—you may have guessed it—the people. I'd be able to deal with the parking lot, the bags, the carts, the in-between, anything if the place were empty. But it is never empty.

Have a look. Here's a lady in her pajamas, meandering aimlessly right in front of the exact item I need. Here is the spandex-clad dude on a speed run, brushing past me and grabbing the last box of raspberry Pop Tarts. *Hello!* A splotchy, wet-faced kid crying for a sugary cereal. And greetings to the family of six taking up the entire width of the aisle and headed right toward me.

Maddening.

Due to COVID, the store even put arrows on the floor, telling everyone which direction to go. It should stay this way for good since having one-way aisles would help the flow of traffic … if anyone actually fucking followed the arrows!

Am I the only one following the arrows? Why is no one following the arrows?

Whenever someone comes toward me, walking against the arrows, I give them the hairy eyeball. Then I look down at the arrow on the ground and look back up at them, my eyebrow slightly raised. *Notice something wrong?* my inquisitive eyebrow asks them. They do not seem to understand. I become angrier.

Okay, that's enough. Everything else about grocery shopping sucks, but I'll spare you the extra details. Checkout sucks, walking the shopping cart to the car and unloading it sucks. Returning the empty shopping cart majorly sucks, getting home and unloading the car absolutely sucks. Realizing I forgot something sucks the big one. How does Cali do this every few days?

My point in telling you all this is, in spite of my supermarket challenges, God *forbid* I substitute anything. Something like, let's say, a certain kind of peanut butter. In the past, if they were out of Skippy Smooth Peanut Butter, I might've actually picked up Skippy Super Chunk Extra Crunchy instead, if they had it. In fact, I'd be psyched about Super Chunk Extra Crunchy instead of Smooth. Extra Crunchy sounds awesome. *Add a little excitement to that PB&J? Yes, please.* We may like it so much that Skippy Super Chunk Extra Crunchy becomes a permanent amendment to the ole shopping list. I'm an innovator, and I deliver.

But I know now that when I get home with the groceries and lay them all out on the kitchen counter, that is when Cali begins her inspection. I see her, sifting through and examining each item; mentally comparing it to the shopping list she wrote and then rewrote because it'd been a little sloppy. Then there's me, mentally and physically exhausted from my journey.

And that's when she says it. "I really appreciate you picking up the groceries …"

"Okay," I say cautiously.

"But you got the wrong peanut butter."

She noticed.

"They didn't have the other, so I got this. Looks good, right?"

"Ella can't eat this kind because she's allergic to anything chunky. She will die if she eats it, so good job, you almost killed your daughter.

That's why we never have chunky-style mashed potatoes. She can only eat smooth foods."

"What?"

"And Ella needed this jar of *smooth* peanut butter for a school project on *smooth things* that is due tomorrow, so I'm really going to need you to go back out, or she isn't going to graduate. Also, quick reminder: You're a bad dad, a terrible shopper, and not a real man."

Not her exact words, but that's pretty much what I hear.

So, for this reason, I did not grab the Skippy Super Chunk Extra Crunchy Peanut Butter at CVS. I called Cali from the car and told her they didn't have what she needed. She asked me if I could go to Super Stop & Shop to get it. Plus, they had called in a *different* prescription that was ready at *that* pharmacy, the one we normally used.

Perfect. You bet. I'm here to help.

I began driving toward our local Stop & Shop, already dreading the experience.

Plus, I still hadn't forgotten that a week ago, when I picked up a prescription at the Stop & Shop Pharmacy, everyone in the pharmacy made fun of me. I'm not kidding. All three employees there joined together and picked on me.

"*Oh*, to what do we owe the pleasure?"

"Yes, the prince has left his castle!"

"Where's Cali? It must be something *really important* if it got *you* out to actually pick up the prescriptions."

Who are these people?

I felt like telling them Cali couldn't make it because she had cancer, just to shut them up and make them feel terrible. I'm not quite that vindictive though. But to my knowledge, this was highly unprofessional pharmacist behavior.

Anyway, this time, the gang of bullying pharmacists must have deduced Cali's condition based on the prescriptions I was filling and the fact that I was there for the second time in a row. I could tell because no one teased me for leaving my "lair." Also, because one of the women who works there—a lovely woman in a white lab coat— came around from behind the partition and approached me. I had seen her before, but to me, she was a piece of furniture. Just another person to avoid or ignore as I navigated the supermarket. She got close and looked up at me, her eyes welling up with tears.

What the fuck?

"How is she?" she asked, her voice quivering.

"How is *who*?" I queried.

"Your wife, Cali." She was pleading now.

Okay, she knows Cali. And she knows Cali is sick. Got it.

I explained Cali was doing well, considering she'd had her first round of treatment last week; she was very tired but no nausea yet.

I knew Cali was here often, but the idea she had connected so strongly with this woman at the pharmacy was perplexing.

"I went through it last year," she informed me.

I was surprised at her candor. I didn't know what to say, so to be polite, I asked her how it was—as if I were asking about a movie she'd seen recently.

She told me about her experience in detail. She'd been able to handle the nausea when she was pregnant, but cancer was different because there wasn't a beautiful baby inside you.

It's something else growing inside you, I thought morbidly.

I told her Cali was the same way. She had loved being pregnant and handled it like a champ.

We talked for a while. There I was, talking and maybe crying a little with Momma Labcoat in the middle of a crowded grocery store.

"She's an amazing lady, your wife. Please send her my love." She could barely get the words out. She would have touched me, if it weren't for COVID. I could tell. She wanted to touch me.

I walked away and, a few moments later, let out an audible sob from behind my mask right near a startled bag boy.

What the actual fuck just happened?

I walk around this planet, dreading every moment and trying to avoid any human interaction like it is a living obstacle course. Conversely, my wife had clearly touched the hearts of random pharmacists, not to mention various others, during her daily life. I was moved, yet ponderous. Who else was Cali touching?

Shut up, you know what I mean.

CHAPTER 14
Bottle It Up

I took Cali in the next morning to get her port inspected. The doctor said it looked good. I could have told her that at home.

I'm not exactly sure what my plan was, but I spent part of the afternoon looking online for photos of strong women. I was trying to find an image that would be motivational to Cali so I could put it on her desk or night table. I don't know. I felt like making a gesture.

I searched "warrior women" and got a bunch of battle-hardened Vikings. "Strong women" resulted mostly in photos of women working out. The internet was too vast to show me what I needed based on a loose description. I was also walking a high wire over a porn vortex with the slightly wrong search term. Finally, I determined I had to think of someone specific. Cali already had a bobble head of RBG on her desk, so that wouldn't work, although it would have been a good one.

How about Serena Williams?

She was a female warrior and mother who fought adversity. Every photo or piece of art I found with Serena had her looking pissed off—but not in a good, fierce-and-ready-to-fight way. More like an I'm-questioning-this-call-and-being-a-bit-of-a-baby way.

I searched female action heroines, historically strong women, sports figures. There was no shortage of strong women in history, sports, and entertainment, but nothing fit perfectly. I gave up.

Really, just a picture of Cali herself would have done the trick. She was turning out to be the strongest woman I could think of.

That afternoon, I was talking to my brother-in-law Aaron. He's married to Cali's sister Shari, and they have three kids who are like siblings to my kids. Aaron and I are like brothers. We've spent that much time together since day one. I'm the same way with Cali's brother Sean. And they all love my brother Bryan. We got lucky that way.

Aaron is a solid dude who would do anything for me. For anyone, really. We've known each other for a long time now and have a pretty good way of communicating. He is a few years older than me, and while there's a slight big-brother vibe, I feel very close to him. I trust him for sure.

Aaron's father, Jack, is cool, but I get the feeling he was old school back in the day. Maybe that's why Aaron seems to have slightly more traditional beliefs about men and women and their respective roles in the world and in relationships.

I didn't say *chauvinistic*. *You* said chauvinistic. I said *slightly more traditional*, and I'm telling you this because it relates to this particular conversation. Also, Aaron's mom, Georgie, had lymphoma. She fought it off for many, many years before she passed.

Anyway, we were on the phone and Aaron asked how I was doing.

So, I told him about how I'd lost my shit when I picked Cali up from that first day of chemo. And how I was a bit of a dick the second day. Maybe I wasn't doing the best job.

After I took him through the rest of my week and how I was feeling a bit overwhelmed, he said, "Wow, that's a lot. I guess it's better that you're telling me instead of burdening Cali though."

I told him no, Cali knew how I felt. We were being very open with each other about our feelings during this whole thing.

He was quiet for a second then said, "When my mom went through it, my dad was like a soldier. He never said a word and just followed his marching orders. He didn't want to take away from what my mom was going through."

I felt a pang of guilt.

At the very same time I was having this conversation, I shit you not, my mother-in law texted me, which was kind of unusual.

How are you doing? she inquired.

I cautiously typed back that I was okay. Some ups and downs, but I was hanging in there.

She wrote back, *Okay, but we need to keep it together for Cali. We need to be strong.*

After careful consideration, I responded, *Of course, totally agree.*

Just one of these two conversations would have gotten me thinking, but both? At the same time? Something was afoot. This family's grapevine was like no other, and now I was imagining them all having an emergency meeting to talk about their friend Gregg.

"He is feeling *emotions* and *telling Cali.*"

"I have to tell you, it's selfish."

Her family always says, "I have to tell you" before they tell you anything for some reason.

"This is about *Cali. He* doesn't have cancer. He's distracting her and needs to suck it up."

"I never liked him."

Just kidding about that last one. Probably.

Now first, these comments about me, which I completely made up, were way out of line. I felt that Cali and I were communicating openly about things, and that was good. Second, I certainly wasn't sucking all the air out of the room with my bellyaching. Not by a long shot ... I hoped. And finally, if I kept my mouth shut and was just straight-faced and stoic, wouldn't Cali think her husband didn't really give a shit? Or have any feelings about her? I was proud of us based on how we'd handled the communications so far. It seemed healthy.

I stewed over the coincidental messages for a bit and then called Aaron back after a while. *Screw it.* I told him about Arlene's text, the overlap with his call, and my suspicions that I was the subject of some family analysis and subsequent disapproval. Okay, fine, I *texted* him all this, but either way.

He told me that was absolutely not the case. Total coincidence between his call and Arlene's text. Also, that probably was not what Arlene had meant, and it was certainly not what he had meant either. He wrote:

I don't think I know what's right or wrong, to be honest. I learned what I learned from my dad. He hid it from everyone—my mom, us kids—so that's I guess how I see it.

He continued: But what you said about being open makes a lot of sense too. I also know you well enough to know that if Cali needs you, you're there. If you think being upset or even crying in front of her is no good, then you won't, and if you judge that it is okay, then you will. You're a smart, good husband and man. I could probably learn a lot from you.

If you know Aaron, that's a lot.

Damn allergies again.

CHAPTER 15
Taking Inventory

I woke up the following Monday morning feeling not fully awake after a restless night. My belly felt extra-large after a weekend of overdrinking and overeating, which is required by law during the early rounds of the March Madness tournament. As a result, I felt heavy and sluggish. I reminded myself to make a doctor's appointment. My blood sugar had been high last time, officially categorizing me as prediabetic. I had dabbled with intermittent fasting, which is supposed to help level that out, but my streak didn't last long, and the past month had seen me back to my normal habits, if not worse. I was frequently getting dizzy and lightheaded, seeing spots before my eyes, and I had a general sense of malaise. I can only explain by saying it felt like I had thick syrup in my veins, which was probably from having actual thick syrup in my veins.

I also had other things on my mind aside from *mywifeissick, mywifeissick, mywifeissick* and my own health concerns. I had a to-do list a mile long that I had just completely ignored. The weather was continuing to warm up, and spring had officially sprung over the weekend. This made me feel a nagging pressure to power-wash the house, spray for bugs, paint the rotted bay window, fix the banged-up border on the garage, reorganize the garage, and cut back the thorny branches that had grown through the fence. I also had to call someone to come spruce up the landscaping, repair my back patio, and look at the AC units. And I needed to put away all the ice-fishing gear still in sleds in the basement since February, replace all the 9-volt batteries in the fire alarms, go through my clothes and throw out anything that didn't fit—which would leave me with two shirts and a sock—look at new outdoor furniture for the deck, get some art to hang on the walls that had been bare since we'd painted a year ago, and so on.

Owning a home is fun.

I also had a backlog of a few hundred work emails, price quotes that were due this week, projects that were in jeopardy if I didn't act soon, and that nagging feeling that any one of my three hundred customers could be unhappy about something without my knowing about it. The imaginary thought that my team at work was secretly irritated and abuzz about my lack of involvement lately, the overall threat of every competitor coming after us, and the potential for our business to be taken away and moved permanently to China was also hanging over me.

I was also thinking about Alix, who'd called crying again this weekend from Tulane. From the amazing city of New Orleans. From the school that was costing me $79,000 a year. Naturally, she was sad about her mom, but she was also feeling insecure and lonely. Her anxiety was acting up, and she didn't know if her boyfriend thought she was annoying. For seventy-nine grand, that freaking school should've thrown a parade for my daughter if she was feeling down; instead, I grew angrier as I heard the construction booming on the other end of the phone that had rocked her dorm since September.

I was also thinking about Hunter, who, as a junior at *the* Ohio State University, probably should have already applied for summer internships many months ago. Here we were, a few days into spring, and nothing. In his defense, he was president of his fraternity and getting straight As. But it would be no fun for me to focus on that. He had sat on completing his résumé, and now that it was finally done, he was dragging his ass on his cover letter. Not to mention he hadn't submitted one single application yet. Whenever I asked him about it, he said he was slammed with schoolwork. And while his grades were great, every time I saw him, he was either shirtless in bed at 2 p.m. or at a toga party or at a Hawaiian-themed party or at a date party or at a *darty* (daytime party) or telling me he'd just binge-watched seven seasons of *New Girl* in a week. I'm no detective, but it seemed like there was a *little* free time in there for the résumé and internship search.

And Ella. Her high school friend group was great one day and having a major rift the next. Girls were breaking off and pairing up and tripling up and quadrupling up, and the only common denominator in this shitty math equation was that Ella seemed to be the one left out. She didn't know what she was going to do this summer, she had made zero progress on her college search (my fault), and everyone else seemed to know exactly where they wanted to apply. She wasn't dating anyone, which was fine with me, but it seemed that everyone else was sowing their wild, young oats. She was nervous about her impending lacrosse tryouts and seemed to have an overwhelming amount of schoolwork.

Plus, all three of my kids had their mom on their minds, and I didn't really know how to help them with that either.

So, as Cali and I drove to her Monday morning doctor appointment for her blood work, I was deep inside my head.

After a while, the silence must have alerted Cali. "What's wrong?" she asked, halfway to the hospital.

"Nothing," I said, thinking of her mom's text.

Good soldier.

CHAPTER 16
The Wig Situation

Today, three generations of women joined together to make a pilgrimage to the holy land of Great Neck, in search of a proper wig for Mrs. Cali Goldman.

I should back up.

From the moment we got the news about Cali, her biggest concern had been losing her hair. I guess having had the hysterectomy just before all this, the resulting concerns about losing her femininity were only magnified by the probability of Cali's impending hair loss. Not to mention her eyebrows and eyelashes as well, most likely. I knew it wasn't vanity or self-indulgence, but I couldn't personally understand her preoccupation with the hair. If faced with cancer, I'd primarily be concerned about, I don't know, dying. I'd also be apprehensive about feeling terrible all the time during treatment. Perhaps I'd even worry about bullying pharmacists. A million other things would concern me before the hair thing. Of course, Cali was indeed concerned about all those other things. But there was a lot of hair talk right out of the gate.

I'd said to her one of those days, "Cali, why are you so worried about losing your hair? As soon as it starts thinning, just shave it, like you're a badass Amazonian warrior. Wear the baldness like a badge of honor."

She'd looked at me as if I had just told her I'd done the dishes. "Are you crazy?" she wanted to know. "I am getting a wig right away before I even lose my hair. There's no way I am going around bald. You are totally misunderstanding what it is going to be like for me."

I'd chalked up my lack of understanding to Cali being the one going through this and not me. Or Cali being a woman and me being a man. Or Cali being smart and me being a moron. Either way, she made it clear: I was out of my element.

A few days in, Cali told me her sister had found the perfect wig woman. She was in Great Neck, Long Island. We do not live near there. This woman was reputed to be the Wonderful Wizard of Wigs though, and Cali was excited. The going rate at Wanda's Wig Emporium is around $3,500. But it's worth it because the wigs are so *real looking*. And made from *real hair*. Oh, by the way, that doesn't include the backup wig that is just hair on the sides so you can wear a baseball cap or a cowboy hat or an astronaut helmet over it. That one is extra.

An appointment had been made immediately for three weeks out. It was right before Passover, and Wigs R Us was very busy before the holidays, so the timing was critical, and the slots were limited. It was hereby decreed that Cali's sister Shari, Cali's mother, and Ella would accompany Cali. Alix would be on standby in New Orleans to be connected via FaceTime at any critical juncture.

I immediately began busting chops about the wig situation. I don't know why it bothered me so much, but pretty much everything does, so I wasn't surprised.

"Cali," I inquired. "Let me ask you something. Do you think it is possible that somewhere between here and Great Neck, there is another wig place that specializes in cancer patients and is worth checking out?"

"No. This place is the best. Any other place is no good." Actual answer.

"Would you like me to look into another place that is, let's say, closer, or, I don't know, less expensive?"

"No. Stop."

This situation suddenly felt familiar to me. I thought back to the time before our wedding. Cali and her mom had everything sorted out and under control. The wedding had already been planned twenty-eight years earlier, but I was too dumb to realize that then.

When it was time for Cali to find a wedding dress, I was excited. There was barely an internet back then. Sure, there was Netscape Navigator. There were only around one hundred thousand websites in 1996 leading up to our wedding, and half of them were text-based. Nothing like we have today. But there was no shortage of bridal magazines to be perused for ideas. *It would be fun!* That was when I learned I wasn't going to be part of this journey. There was a place in Brooklyn called Kleinfeld Bridal. Cali, her mother, and her sister were going together. It was all very *exclusive*, and each visit and subsequent fitting appointment was a major event. There was something tribal about it.

I was jealous. As a result, I began to lash out. My life already felt a little out of control. I was only twenty-four, a mere babe, although I didn't realize it then. Cali is four years older than me, which, at the time, was pretty cool. I was marrying a *woman* who had already been a kindergarten teacher for several years. She was a real person.

So, feeling out of control and scared, what do we do? We lash out. Well, at least I do.

I became difficult during the wedding planning. During our visit to the venue to review the music, the coordinator asked if there were any songs we didn't like. I requested we skip the hora; it was too old-fashioned. Cali's parents just stared at me and probably gave the caterer an imperceptible shake of the head.

Don't mind him, he's a buffoon.

"Gregg, would you like to see the invitation?"

Of course, I would. Let me have a peek. "Oh, I thought the font would be different. Can we change it?"

Silence. Shock. Disgust, probably.

Did I mention that Cali's parents paid for almost everything? Yes, it was going to be the wedding Cali and her mom had fantasized about, and I'd be lying if I said I had ever given it a moment's thought before then. I was just being a pain in the ass, which, of course, caused arguments between me and Cali and probably some choice words from her parents about this young, dumb fool with no money and a lot of opinions.

In retrospect, I *wish* I could go back and do it differently. I don't mean I wouldn't get married. I mean I would just show up and shut up. I was clearly acting out because I felt scared and out of control. It could have been a much nicer experience all around if I'd realized what I was really doing.

This wig situation had that same out-of-control feeling. I was scared and felt like my life was spiraling, so I imposed myself on a nice moment between the women in the family. I had learned nothing.

No!

I *would* learn from the error of my ways. I *would* "show up and shut up." I *would not* make the same mistake twice. Or thrice, even, because I had done this when each of my three kids were born too. I let go of trying to control the wig situation.

Plus, Cali's parents had told her they were paying for it.

★ ★ ★

The wig thing went well. Cali and Ella didn't get home until almost 8 p.m. It was a long and, apparently, emotional process right out of the gate. Everyone was reportedly crying at various times, and the woman there had been amazing, helpful, and gracious. Cali came home with one full wig and the special hat one. She placed each one on its own foam bust on the shelf in her closet. They freaked me out.

Let me briefly take you back to Florida, 1982. I was ten years old, and it was Christmas break at Harold and Esther Kazdin's—my mother's parents'—house at Del Boca Vista in Delray Beach. For some reason all the adults were out on this rainy day and left us kids home alone. But my brother and I had a plan. Bryan, my younger brother by three years, was giddy with excitement as we tiptoed quietly into my grandfather's small walk-in closet. That inner sanctum smelled of stale cigarettes and aftershave.

Harold had smoked heavily back then. Later, when the doctor told him to quit or suffer the consequences, he kept a pack in a toolbox in the garage. Every evening, he'd wander into the garage under the pretense of some errand, where he would light up and take two puffs. He kept the hedge clippers on the shelf and would clip the cigarette to save the rest for next time. It must have taken him three days to finish a full cigarette. He'd come back in, reeking of smoke, and never say a word. If it ever came up in a discussion, he'd say he quit years ago. We all knew exactly what he was up to back then.

Anyway, Florida. Adults gone. Giddy tiptoeing into the closet. And there on Grandpa Harold's shelf sat a foam head, not unlike the ones Cali came home with. Perched atop that white, featureless head lay the holy grail for idiot kids on a rainy day: Harold Kazdin's toupee.

"Touch it!" my brother squealed—daring me, but simultaneously begging.

We got up close. We put our hands out like little claws, drawing nearer, creeping closer. Our fingers wiggled, like we were witches approaching a cauldron. Bryan pushed my hand, and it touched the faux hair. My hand snapped back, but the threshold had been crossed. I picked up the toupee after removing the two pins holding it in place. The inside was some kind of rubbery foreign material that would surely stick to a bald scalp. The outside was hair, different shades of gray and silver to match what was remaining on our grandfather's head. It oddly felt real and fake at the same time. The hair was coarse and stiff. I put it on and looked in the mirror. It looked like a gray helmet on my small head but still somehow made me feel older. I puffed out my chest and said some things an older person would say.

"Esther, we need to do the taxes!"

My brother giggled with absolute delight, his pre-braced teeth spread out like wild Chiclets, his chicken legs dancing back and forth in his knee-high, white-striped socks and short shorts. "Let me try! Let me try!" he pleaded, putting his arms out to receive the forbidden toy.

We'd messed about with the hairpiece for an hour or so, putting it back as carefully as we could, but there was no way it was exactly the way Grandpa Harold had it.

Later that night, we heard Harold's raised voice coming from his bedroom. My mother's muffled voice could be heard as well—reasoning, explaining. I can only imagine he wanted to tear us each a new one, and my mother intervened. She succeeded in saving our butts because we never heard a word about it.

I never forgot that foreign, forbidden feeling the foam head and fake hair gave me. Well, actually, I had forgotten it until I peeked into Cali's closet that night, and it all came back.

I had no desire to put her wig on and play with it though.

CHAPTER 17
A Shiny New Object

How do people have pools? They're incredibly expensive, require almost a year of planning and paperwork before installation, and everyone I know says they're a pain in the ass to maintain.

I want one.

Cali has always wanted a pool too. Many years ago, we'd had some cash for a project, but it was only enough to either finish the basement or put in a pool. At the time, the basement was the best decision for us. It became a bit of a man cave for me, but the kids were older then, and it was a great place for them to hang out with their friends. Also, the kids were away at camp during the summer, so it just never made sense to put in a pool.

The last few summers, though, the kids have been around more. Cali and I have spent many sweaty afternoons on the deck, fantasizing about a pool but always dismissing the idea due to expense and hassle. Now, between COVID, Cali being sick, and Cali reminding me repeatedly she'd *really* love a pool, I was leaning toward saying, "Screw it."

I did some digging online and found ten reputable pool companies in the area. So, on Friday, March 26 at 9 a.m., I reached out to each with either a voicemail or email. The message was the same: I wanted to know if there was any chance in hell of getting a pool installed for use this summer. Then I went back to work.

During the day, the responses began trickling in via phone call or email. By that afternoon, nine of the ten had replied. There was no chance in hell I could have a pool in for this summer. In fact, I couldn't have one installed by the fall, and they were already backed up for spring of '22. COVID had everyone scrambling to put in pools, decks, patios, outdoor heaters, home offices, and probably some really cool underground bunkers.

I had all but given up when the phone rang that evening. It was Jim from Pooling Around or something to say, sure, he could get it done for me. How about he sends his son, Jim Junior, out there to see me tomorrow? But first, how about he takes me through everything that needs to be done and what it will cost? Ten minutes in and the fog started rolling into the corners of my mind. Fifteen minutes and I gave up trying to take notes or add up the cost of everything he was listing. I can't count that high anyway.

Still, I told him to go ahead and send Jim Junior my way. Cali wanted a pool.

★★★

Jim Junior from Pooling Around came by and brought John from Gonnascrewya Construction. We walked around the backyard and talked about what I was looking for. Then we huddled around the locker-style freezer I have in the garage. It is supposed to be for deer meat, but I had struck out this season, so it was filled with frozen pizzas and sadness. Today, it served as a desk.

I didn't want to bring these two into the house because I was trying not to expose Cali, who was immunocompromised and unvaccinated. But it was cold out this morning, and I was losing patience fast as Jim Junior struggled to do some addition and subtraction to figure out the total.

Things had started well though. We wound up laughing about my crazy friend Dan, who had recommended these guys. When Dan gave me their info, he said, "Goldy, whatever you think this is gonna cost, double it."

Great.

Jim Junior and I laughed as he told me a story about when he had installed Dan's pool. Dan's neighbors were incredibly difficult. Joel and Carol were always complaining, no matter what Dan and his wife, Amy, did. At one point two years ago, they'd confronted Dan's son, Henry, and his friends face-to-face for making too much noise one afternoon as they played ball outside. It was 3 p.m. Dan almost murdered them, as would I.

Well, Joel and Carol showed up just as the pool guys started digging. Their phones were out, recording video, and Dan came out, asking what their problem was. The wife just kept recording as the husband dialed the town of Somers right in front of Dan, asking who he could speak to if he wanted to check that permits were in order.

When Joel finally hung up, he and Dan had words. Things got heated. The two project managers, Jim Junior and John, got involved, and the rest of the work crew began to approach, curious about the hubbub.

Dan continued arguing as everyone gathered around. "And another thing, Joel. You're really going to stand here and tell me—"

The wife took a step forward, finger pointed in the air, and opened her mouth to speak.

Dan didn't miss a beat. "Shut the fuck up, Carol!"

Suddenly, *everyone* shut the fuck up. Carol. Joel. Jim Junior. John. The crew. Birds.

When they snapped out of it, Joel just muttered to himself as he and Carol walked away.

Jim Junior and John were having a good old time telling me this story, and I was having a good time hearing it. They couldn't believe what Dan had said, but they were even more impressed that Dan didn't get punched. I hadn't thought about that, but they were right. Crazy.

So, we had some laughs. Then Jim Junior finished his math problem and showed me the result.

I stopped laughing right away and somberly wrote him a check.

CHAPTER 18

The Fortunate Son

I spent the next morning writing my son's cover letter.

At this point, Hunter was a junior in the Fisher School of Business at *the* Ohio State University. He was majoring in marketing, which he had selected based on his lifelong passion for the subject. No, wait, it wasn't that. It was an easier course load than accounting or finance, that was it.

To his credit, he was also double-minoring in economics and, get this, the video game industry. It sounds like a joke, but I read recently that the video game industry is surpassing the North American sports and entertainment industries *combined*. So, when Hunter told me about his desire to minor in video games, I made him a deal. *Double* minor in both video games *and* economics. It just sounded less flaky to me from a résumé standpoint, even though the kid probably knows better.

The summer of junior year is known to those who are serious about a career as Internship Time. Résumés and applications are normally in by November for that following summer. The competition is fierce to garner a coveted spot where one can gain valuable experience in their chosen field. With last summer having been a total COVID clusterfuck, this summer saw a higher number of applicants than usual, looking to cut their teeth and actually leave their house if they were lucky.

It was the end of March though, not November. Way *past* November, if my calculations were correct. When I would bring up the subject, Hunter would say he needed to "polish his résumé." I told him to get on over to the career counseling office and polish away. They certainly had the resources to help him. That was one of the reasons he'd chosen OSU.

I thought back to our campus tour when Hunter was a prospective student. We had stood in the center of a perfectly manicured green quad as the tour guide whispered sweet nothings into our ears. We were surrounded by the modern yet collegiate brick architecture of the Fisher School of Business facilities bordering the quad, gleaming with new windows and festooned with the names of wealthy alumni donors. I imagined Hunter lying there in the vibrant green grass in between classes, reading something by Dale Carnegie, a beautiful female classmate next to him, staring at that little curl of hair that twirled down over Hunter's forehead as she adjusted her plaid skirt and pretended to study.

We entered the main building where they showed us endless rows of Apple computers and 3D printers. "And if you'll just step this way, you will see our bustling career counseling office." OSU's staff would work with each individual student to find the field that was right for them. Then, through a revolutionary interview training program, required for all business students before they could schedule an actual job interview through the school, said students would become better prepared than anyone to demonstrate their qualifications. I could see Hunter in a blue pinstripe suit and a tasteful tie, learning the ins and outs of the interview technique.

My biggest weakness? Well, sir, I tend to care too much. Ha, ha, ha. Yes, it's a curse.

With the help of the Fisher School of Business, Hunter would discover his passion in wind-powered digital currency. He'd learn how to crush an interview and create the very first holographic résumé, which would not only demonstrate that he's an innovator but would also show him in 4D action as a leader and worker. Without telling anyone, he'd take the red-eye to Palo Alto on his own and camp out until Elon Musk agreed to see him. The rest would be history. It would only be a matter of time before he'd appear on the cover of *YBM* (*Young Billionaire Magazine*), and at age twenty-seven, he'd buy his parents a sprawling estate in San Diego—the first of many incredible gifts to us as a "thank you" for the support.

Sorry, what? I zoned out there for a minute.

After several inquiries, Hunter had finally agreed to send me a copy of his résumé so I could polish that turd for him. I couldn't stand waiting any longer for him to do it, and the stakes were too high for me to teach him a lesson and let him fail by not doing anything. What he sent me might have been written in crayon, but he did get his name right. I kid, I kid. It was fine. I punched it up, typed a bunch of suggestions into an email, and hit send. Then I waited.

Weeks passed, and when I asked him to send an updated résumé for the umpteenth time, Hunter explained again that he was "extremely busy." I suppose I'm a skeptic, but I asked how busy he could be since I knew for a fact that he slept until 2 p.m. almost every day and partied hard almost every night.

Then he explained it, and I felt bad.

"Dad, just because I keep different hours than you doesn't mean I'm not active for the same, if not greater, amount of time. It's taking everything in my power to keep solid As in all my classes. And remember, I've been president of the fraternity this past year, which has been a great experience but a lot of responsibility. *And* you've said on numerous occasions how important it is for me to have a balance between work and play while I'm at college."

The kid should be a politician.

I thought back to my booze-filled, five-year bender at Michigan State University. I wouldn't trade those fuzzy and probably great memories for anything. Then I pictured Hunter graduating in a year and going off to work. Marching onto the subway like every other corporate drone, just trying to earn enough money to pay rent and afford a few beers on the weekend. Depressing. No wonder he was putting it off.

So, I typed up his résumé. And today, I typed his cover letter. It was all real information; I was just helping him out, like an assistant would. And he tweaked the cover letter to reflect his own voice. Probably.

Was I doing him a disservice? I imagined how it might be if things continued in this manner. Maybe something like this:

"Hey, son, when are you going to make an honest woman of that beautiful brain surgeon you've been dating?"

"I don't know, Dad. I've been really busy."

"Well, let me help you out, son."

I head over to the hospital where Hunter's girlfriend emerges in her scrubs. She has just finished a nine-hour surgery. I get down on one knee and tell her everything I think Hunter probably feels about her. That I think he can't wait to spend the rest of his life with her, but I'm sure he'll tell her in his own words at some point when he's not so busy.

She accepts.

We don't kiss. That would be weird.

Fast-forward a few years, and I'm playing catch with his son as Hunter takes a nap in a hammock nearby, exhausted from work. I just got him a promotion, you see, and the pressure has really ratcheted up. He's worried I'm not keeping up with the workload, and that's really stressing him out. Plus, I haven't even fixed the garbage disposal like I promised, and I'm only halfway through writing his acceptance speech for an honorary doctorate from OSU.

Once again, I'm just kidding. The kid is under a lot of pressure. Really.

CHAPTER 19
Round Two: Ding. Ding.

On March 29, 2021, Cali began her second round of treatment. The nurses said the side effects would accelerate from here on in, meaning the nausea and hair loss and general discomfort would multiply. Cali had only felt nauseous twice so far. She is normally a *tough guy* when it comes to medication in general and would rather suffer through a simple headache than take something for the pain, which makes zero sense to me. We have the same argument every time it comes up, and she has yet to offer a logical explanation.

"I have such a headache," Cali laments.

"Take something," I suggest, always the problem-solver.

"No, I'm fine," she says paradoxically.

What the fuck? I think to myself. Or sometimes say out loud.

Luckily, the nurses had warned Cali if she felt even a tiny bit of nausea coming on, then she needed to take the medication immediately because it would otherwise get much worse and more difficult to get relief. So, if she felt a little queasy, Cali took the chewable pill, and the discomfort went away. I made her promise to take it if she felt anything. She agreed.

The first time around, *R* day had taken eight hours and included a halftime show featuring the *Cali*bama Shakes. But this time, the nurses cranked up the drip rate even more, and Cali did just fine. I had gone home to work, and Cali was finished after just five hours. The tiny circular pickup/drop-off area was full of vehicles, so I swung around and exited the lot, planning to park on the street until Cali was ready. There were no spots, but I saw a hydrant and parked there. I figured if a cop pulled up, or if there were an actual fire, I could pull right out quickly.

Besides, I had become very good at identifying fire hydrants lately, having to pick them out in a lineup of photos to prove to the internet I was not a robot. I am also great at recognizing crosswalks and traffic lights. I do get stressed out, though, if a small part of the traffic light is bleeding into another square on the segmented photo. Do I click that square or not? It's technically part of a traffic light, but does the computer know that? Can't they come up with a less confusing method to prove I am not a robot? More importantly, *why* do I have to prove I am not a robot? If phase one of the evil robot plan was to misdiagnose people with lymphoma, phase two must be to randomly order a bunch of shit on the internet.

Damn you, robots!

★ ★ ★

At work, I tend to do the same thing I do in my personal life: I don't get super close to anyone—to my co-workers, I mean; with my customers, it's a different story.

I've gotten much better over time, though, having been at the same place for over twenty-five years. But for many of those years, people probably figured I wasn't the worst guy in the world but also not the best. And for many of those years, I'd say they were right. I never cared about anything but getting my work done. If someone was in my way, I would plow right through them. I convinced myself I was the only one who cared or was capable.

Over the last fifteen years, though, I'd smartened up. I saw things differently when I had kids, my own personal issues, and a mortgage to pay. I realized it was terrible to talk badly about a co-worker without giving them a chance. I also realized most people probably had inaccurate judgments about me, so chances were I was wrong about them too. So I stopped being shady and started keeping my mouth shut. In fact, if I had a problem, I would speak directly to the person involved. I would explain that this information was not going to anyone else, that I knew they worked hard and cared about things, but something about the company procedures or their level of support was an issue, and I wanted to help them. I began to find that when someone realized I wasn't the enemy and was just being a stand-up guy trying to work things out directly, they tended to want to help instead of quietly resenting and plotting against me.

This wasn't a change in *technique*. That is an important distinction. That would be calculated and manipulative. I had a legitimate change in mindset and a newfound appreciation for everyone who busted their ass.

It doesn't help that since I'm in sales, I'm in front of customers much more than my co-workers. And my job dictates that I'm always the one screaming internally about meeting deadlines and advocating for the customer.

I'm also not one for small talk, which may seem strange for a salesperson. When I first started working, I was astounded by the amount of time being "wasted" by casual conversation. People would hang around each other's cubes, shooting the shit, and it drove me bonkers. *How dare they use company time to get to know each other personally?* And if someone cornered me for a convo, forget about it. I wanted out of there right away. Why on Earth would I waste time talking to these people when I could be getting my work done so I could get the hell out of there? It didn't make sense. Later, when I got into sales, the feeling only magnified since I spent so much time schmoozing with customers and had no time or energy for my own co-workers.

Take my sales coordinator, Kamini. I've worked with her for over twenty years, and I'm proud to say I know nothing about her. That's not entirely true. Maybe twice a year, we have an actual personal conversation; the rest of the year, I'm just cranky and all business.

I remember when I started working with Kamini. She was friends with Mitchell's former assistant, who had referred her, so we brought Kamini on as a temp. That first year, Mitchell's former assistant and

Kamini would laugh at all my stupid jokes. The first time they met Cali, they were eager to tell her how great I was.

"Oh my God, Cali, you must be laughing *all the time* at home. Gregg is *so funny.*"

Cali cocked her head, looking at them both quizzically. "He's an idiot," she responded, straight-faced.

Now, years later, Kamini does not find me amusing either, and if new customers ask about me, she will inform them, "He's an idiot."

As a result, though, even after all these years, between my general distaste of idle chitchat and overall borderline sociopathic personality, I still occasionally feel like a bit of an outsider at work. But I've also really grown to appreciate a bunch of people.

That was what made it even more moving when word about Cali had spread at my place of employment, and I started getting phone calls. I had expected these guys to show me as much care as I had showed them over the years—hardly any. That wasn't the case though. Call after call came in, and one was more moving than the next. I also realized that any one of these people could have a terrible situation going on at home of which I was completely unaware. Another experience that made me want to be a better person.

★ ★ ★

Everything had gone smoothly with Cali's treatment, so she was ready to roll by the time I got back there. I picked her up, and eventually we pulled into our driveway to a pile of packages on the front steps. Packages were pouring in now as word spread about Cali to customers, friends, and family. We had more blankets than we knew what to do with. Blankets are a popular gift for someone with cancer. I suppose the idea is that the recipient will often be cold during or after treatment. Or frequently lying around on the couch. Both were accurate assessments in Cali's case. The large child in me wanted to build a giant fort.

In addition to blankets, food was the other common gift. We received gift cards for meal delivery services like GrubHub and DoorDash and Uber Eats. All these cute names made me want to start a delivery company called Food Dude or Fry Guy. Even better were the gourmet food boxes or deliveries straight from well-known restaurants. We received a cooler from Zabar's—the famous New York City food emporium—filled with authentic Jewish delicacies just in time for Passover, including potato latkes, chunky applesauce, nova lox, and matzoh ball soup. We had a great meal from that package, which, oddly enough, had come from Ella's friend and her Italian family. Impressive.

Another food gift of note was from one of Alix's roommates' family. They are from Chicago and sent incredible deep-dish pizzas straight from the famous Lou Malnati's. To be honest, I've never heard of the famous Lou Malnati's, or any other famous Chicago pizzeria, for that matter. I spent one drunken haze of a weekend in Chicago in 1994 and might have had some pizza. I know Chicago is known for deep-dish though. Anyway, the pizza was amazing.

We received more lobster roll kits, gourmet popcorn tins, and incredible cookies, including my new favorites from a small shop in Plainview. These cookies had corn flakes and marshmallows inside; sounds weird but tastes so good. Just nuke them first for thirty seconds. Trust me.

It was particularly touching to receive a gift from a customer. In what can sometimes be a one-sided relationship, it warmed my heart to accept what I saw as a symbol of true friendship.

Between all the food being sent, and the Meal Train being in full force, we were eating pretty well—at least I was. Cali and Ella were less excited about these things. And it seemed as though the people who were sending gifts only knew what I'd like to eat, not necessarily what Cali might have wanted.

It was fine with me, but there was a problem: My initial motivation to get healthy when Cali first got sick was slowly fading, and all this grub and hub was not helping.

CHAPTER 20
The Theory of Evolution

I received three pieces of news on the third day of Cali's second round. News that normally wouldn't have affected me the way it had if I weren't so hypersensitive from everything going on with my wife.

First, I got a call from a customer named Quentin. He is a young packaging developer training under an old-school pro. It had been a wild two years for him as he adjusted to the fast-paced, high-stakes, glamorous world of cosmetic packaging.

When you start a new job, I'd say you get a four-month grace period. During that first four months, you can screw anything up, admit you don't know anything, and lean on being new. After that, you get two or three months when your employer starts saying things like, *Remember I showed you that? Or, No, you're not getting it.* After that, all bets are off. You either get it, or people start talking. *Maybe he's not cut out for this.*

Quentin was pushing the limits of that new employee aptitude timeline, and I suspected people were beginning to talk. On top of everything, he's a *low* talker, which is fine, but between the low volume and his general timid demeanor, it was tough to understand everything he said. I could see how people might get irritated, and normally I would've steamrolled right over him. But with my newfound ability to have human feelings, I felt for him. He's a good guy. If he got the hang of things, I knew he'd be great to work with, so I'd been trying to help him out. He knew that if he got stuck or forgot something or was preparing to go into a meeting, he could call me and I'd coach him a bit. I had grown fond of him, and lately he seemed to be getting it a little more.

When Quentin called me, sounding very excited and nervous, I was worried they had finally let him go. It turned out, he was calling to say his new wife was pregnant, and he wanted to tell me personally. He was so proud. I was so moved he was calling me specifically, and I got pretty choked up. It was a nice start to the day.

Secondly, that evening, while Ella, Cali, and I were eating dinner at our little snack tables in the family room and watching *The Great British Baking Show*, I received a text from a customer. He knew I was close with one of my very first customers, Patty F., who'd had a family tragedy. Patty, whom I'll never forget, had been one of the first people to put me at ease during my terrifying first year of sales. I remember sitting across from her in her Long Island office, nervously shifting in my seat and going over a quote for a project in way too much detail.

Mercifully, she stopped me after a while with her Long Island accent. "Listen, cowboy, what does any of this mean anyway? We're all gonna be gone one day, right? You need to relax. Your pricing is good. Don't sell it so hard."

I would have broken my back to help her out after that.

Well, her twenty-six-year-old son had died. My informant said he didn't know the cause.

I paused the show and began crying, which scared the shit out of Cali and Ella. It surprised me too. Normally, I would have just read the text and kept eating and watching, maybe thinking, *Damn, that's rough.* I wouldn't say a word about it until I would mention Patty later to Cali as the woman whose son died two years ago.

"You never told me that," Cali would say.

"Of course I did," I would say incorrectly.

With everything going on with Cali, I sat and imagined what poor Patty must be going through. The shock, grief, and anger she must be experiencing all rippled through me, causing an actual physical response. I told Cali and Ella the cowboy story, along with some others that demonstrated what a good soul Patty is. I couldn't continue watching the show, and I wasn't hungry anymore. That second part was shocking to everyone but true. I got up and paced around for a while, thinking about things.

Not an hour later, I got a text from Kamini. Her brother-in-law had died unexpectedly in India, and she was leaving in the morning to go be with her sister. Once again, I normally would have processed this differently. Kamini's brother-in-law was a distant extra in my movie. A character who had barely minor implications in my own script. I normally would've expressed condolences and been irritated that I had to cover for Kamini over the course of the next week.

And wasn't she scheduled to be on vacation the following week? Yes, I remember her telling me they had decided to go to Aruba since they were all vaccinated. Were they still going?

Instead, I thought about Kamini's sister. I imagined everything she was going through, losing her husband. And Kamini, getting the news, losing someone she cared about. What would it be like if I lost a brother-in-law? It would be an absolute catastrophe. I pictured Kamini telling her daughter, Alysha, the sad news, then booking flights and thinking of a million things before she traveled alone across the globe, including worrying how her idiot boss—me—would react to her being out.

I told Kamini to do whatever she had to and take however long she needed to be there for her sister. I would have said that anyway, but I actually meant it this time. I got choked up again, thinking of Kamini alone on that plane.

Great. I was rapidly evolving from a guy who didn't give a shit about anything to a guy who openly wept about everything.

Time out.

I think you see where this is going, and we know each other well enough to cut the horseshit. Well, you know me well enough. You've been kind of quiet, to be honest.

There's a theme developing. Are you seeing it? I am sensing the formation of a character arc for our protagonist, the ruggedly handsome and slightly overweight curmudgeon. He generally avoids people. His marriage is fine but could use a little spark. His wife is amazing but underappreciated. His kids used to find him enthralling and now not so much. This poor S.O.B. who was previously heading down a dark road finds a fresh appreciation for life, from—of all things—his wife's cancer diagnosis and subsequent treatment.

Our hero emerges from his shell as he begins to see the good in people as a result of their outpouring of affection for him and his family. He gains a newfound respect for his wife as he realizes all the incredible, selfless things she does for him, his family, and others. He gets his large ass in the gym and stops boozing and eating so much, having learned the importance of health and the fragility of life. He has now learned that life is fleeting, and he had better get healthy for his kids so he can stick around long enough to enjoy his grandkids. He learns to love himself, others, various animals. He no longer hates being in public and begins giving back to the community, living a life more focused on service to his fellow man. Our guy is no longer irritated by the asshole in front of him in line at the market, whose mask is sitting on his upper lip right under his nostrils, barely covering his miserable, hairy piehole. He dives into his job with fresh aplomb, finding fulfillment and resulting financial success. His wife beats the absolute shit out of cancer, and they live life to the fucking fullest, traveling and making new friends, touching people's lives all over the goddamn globe.

Sounds incredible!

We'll see. Not sure he's got it in him ….

CHAPTER 21
Summer Lovin'

I rolled over so I was facing away from the window. Since we had changed the clocks, and with the spring days getting longer, morning light had been leaking through the blinds these last few days. It wasn't the light that stirred me though. It was the second flush.

The first flush hit my subconscious while I slept. It was not unusual for Cali to run to the bathroom early morning, and normally it barely registers. My *whooshing* sleep apnea mask makes me feel like a drunken astronaut and tends to cover most outside noises. But hearing the immediate second flush somewhere in dreamland signaled the lizard part of my brain that said, *Something is unusual. Wake up!*

I stirred, half-awake as Cali padded back to bed. That was when I remembered.

The doctor told Cali to flush twice.

They were pumping so much poison into Cali that her urine could be toxic to me if there were some remaining in the bowl after only one flush. It could splash up onto me and, I don't know, melt my legs or burn my dick off. I pictured myself standing at the toilet, looking like the Nazi from *Raiders of the Lost Ark*—but from the waist down.

As Cali settled back into bed, I thought about that and was suddenly wide awake.

What were they doing to her? What was happening inside her?

I rolled over and leaned on my left elbow so I could study my wife, who was already asleep again. Or she was ignoring me and pretending to be asleep. Cali had accumulated a collection of cute pajamas since she was diagnosed. This morning, she lay there in soft cotton pink pajamas, and she looked like a tiny little girl. Her covers were kicked off as usual, and I was astounded at how small she had become.

I told you Cali is barely five foot one, but she always gave a taller appearance thanks to her big personality. It also helped that she always wore giant platform shoes or high heels. She told me recently she had been at her heaviest a year before her diagnosis. We looked back at photos from that year, and she seemed like a different person; the difference was so stark. Cali also takes great care of her appearance and grooming. She is not vain; she just likes to look nice. She gets her nails done regularly. And gets her hair colored every three weeks, just before the skunk stripe appears, replacing her dark-brown roots. Her eyebrows are tweezed. The rogue chin hair is promptly plucked. Cali's makeup is simple but perfectly enhances her complexion to create a healthy glow. Her eyeliner and mascara make her green eyes pop. I remember the first time seeing those eyes, and I often wonder if people who meet her now get hypnotized like I had then, in the summer of 1993.

As a youth, I spent my summers at a sleepaway camp in Massachusetts, where my mother and father ran the waterfront. Later, I became a counselor and waterski instructor. Then, for two summers, I saved my more challenging college classes for the first summer term in East Lansing. I worked at home for the remainder of those summers at odd jobs ranging from loading shipping containers in the July heat to selling children's clothing at Macy's, competing with a school of angry, old sharks who'd worked there for years.

Then I turned twenty. I knew that summer was going to be my last truly free one. The following summer I'd be serving a mandatory internship through the packaging engineering program at Michigan State University. And the following summer, with any luck, I'd have a full-time job in my field of study. I decided I wanted to have one last summer spent in that idyllic camp setting. The camp I had attended and worked at was all boys, and that wasn't going to cut it for my last hurrah. I also hadn't parted ways with that place on the best of terms. Mainly because I was a seventeen-year-old horndog who was more interested in sneaking over to the all-girls camp across the lake at night than being alert enough to safely operate a speedboat with a fragile young child attached to it by day. I knew my tenure had concluded late in the summer when I walked back to my bunk one morning at 7 a.m., as I often did, still drunk and soaking wet just as the reveille bugle blared over the loudspeakers to wake the camp. This time, though, my group leader stood there on my bunk steps, arms folded and daring me to crawl into bed. He ratted me out that afternoon. I didn't blame him.

My brother had worked at a coed sleepaway camp in Pennsylvania with his high school buddy the summer before. He was going back in '93, and I decided to forego my desire to teach waterskiing since they didn't have an open spot in that department. I'd just work as a general counselor so I could spend time with Bryan.

At the time, I was a lean, strapping—dare I say—handsome young fellow. It's all been downhill since then. Scratch that. It's all fallen straight off a cliff since then. Anyway, because of my summer class, I showed up four days into Counselor Orientation week and was warmly welcomed as the "new guy." Four days at camp is like an eternity, so everyone not only knew each other, but in some cases many had already hooked up and ended full relationships. I spent a lot of time being introduced that first week. My co-counselor, Bull, was a veteran there and gave me the skinny on anyone I met or anything I needed to know.

"She's a psycho, stay away."

"That guy is a freak. He dated a sixteen-year-old camper last summer."

"Don't eat the tuna."

Helpful intel, to say the least.

A week later, I felt settled in. We sat in the crowded social hall for the camp's traditional Fourth of July show. It was a mixed bag of skits and inside jokes I didn't totally understand, but I tried to keep up.

I was losing interest fast and entertaining myself by flicking the ear of a camper on the bench in front of me. That was when the bunny hopped out on stage. The show had been progressing through the seasons and, here they were, in spring. And there she was, the bunny. Somehow, I hadn't seen or met her yet. This girl, woman really, now that I think about it, was dressed like a cute little bunny. Well, she had cutoff jean shorts and a white V-neck T-shirt, so it was more of an abstract artistic representation. She did have white bunny ears, and a cute fluffy tail, and she had a little bunny nose with whiskers painted on her face.

Her face …

Just like her smooth legs coming out of those short jean shorts, her face was tan and perfect. Framed by her long, dark-brown hair, her green eyes pierced right though me as she performed. I could swear she was looking right at me, although I was two-thirds of the way back in an auditorium of at least four hundred people. I don't know how well she sang because I could no longer hear. Her perfect, bright-white teeth practically glowed. The rest of the world blurred out. I couldn't see anything else. I was smitten.

I leaned over to Bull as I pushed the two pubescent thirteen-year-olds in between us out of my way. "Who's the bunny?" I asked, my eyes not moving from the stage.

He leaned closer and whispered urgently, "Stay away from her, dude. That's Big Al's daughter."

That got my attention. I looked over at him and he nodded, frowning and shrugging knowingly. *Sorry, buddy.*

Big Al was the director and part owner of this place, and from what I'd heard, he was not to be fucked with.

That is going to be a problem, I thought.

A few hours later, I sat with my campers on the bleachers by the basketball court. It was evening activity, and some of them were playing a loose pickup game. I was coaching.

"Elbow him in the ribs!" I advised expertly.

Just then, the bunny entered my field of vision. Her bunny accessories were gone, but I still managed to recognize her, mostly because I memorized everything about her and had been on a desperate search for her since that afternoon's show. She happened to be walking toward the courts. I had never seen her before, and now I was seeing her twice in the same day. I later learned it was no coincidence. The bunny had noticed me, too, and conveniently had something to take care of in the vicinity of the basketball courts. By "something," I mean absolutely nothing.

Either way, as she approached from afar, we locked eyes. She walked closer, and we held each other's gaze, deeply. I felt like a snake being charmed. I heard a kid go down, his sweaty, shirtless, hairless torso wetly slapping the basketball court as he grunted in pain. I ignored it.

The bunny walked from one end of the court to the other where I was sitting on the bleachers. We were locked in so deep that I was surprised she didn't trip or bump into anyone. This would have been an uncomfortable amount of eye contact if it were anyone else. But in those few seconds, we connected. We looked at each other and sent matching messages: *I am into you, and you are into me. We are about to meet and roar snarl growl.*

The bunny introduced herself, saying she didn't think we'd met yet. I feigned ignorance and said I didn't think we'd met either, but I sure was glad we were meeting now. I can be quite a cunning linguist. She smiled, showing those perfect pearly whites. We talked for a while. There was an undercurrent of electricity from the things not being said. I don't remember our conversation, but then again, I didn't have the normal amount of blood in my head at the time. It was busy elsewhere. Hey, I was young and full of life.

The bunny said her name was Cali, which seemed perfect to me too. *Cali.* Fresh, tan, sunny, unique. Cali told me her job that summer was giving tours to prospective families, so I figured she would have a lot of free time and keys to every building in camp, if you get my drift. She was filling in at waterskiing tomorrow, though, during someone's day off. Maybe I'd swing by, I mentioned nonchalantly.

The next morning, before breakfast, when the kids had to choose their elective activities, I stood in the middle of the bunk and declared, "You're all fucking going waterskiing today!"

So that was how we met. We wound up having one of those magical summers. Each day, we would get so excited when we saw each other.

We were more than happy to just talk, be around each other, and flirt. We'd all go out to the local pub at night and get shitfaced. My little bro was with me, and we accumulated a great crew. After the bar, we'd return to camp and check in at midnight, returning to our bunks. Then Cali and I would sneak out and lay on a hill by the lake or use those keys I knew she had. We would talk about everything and kiss each other under the summer moonlight.

There was not a bad day or night that entire summer.

I looked over at Cali now, remembering those amazing times. She was sleeping on her back with the covers kicked off and her pink PJs hanging loosely off her shrunken body. Her body was even smaller now than the summer I'd met her. Her skin, which always looked tan, was pale. It sagged in some places. Her hip bones poked out through her pajamas, accentuating her concave belly. Her breasts had flattened, and as my gaze moved up to her face, I could see the port tube protruding from her neck, like some alien vein. The skin by Cali's jawline was drawn tight, and her cheeks looked hollow in the pale morning light. Cali's eyes darted back and forth rapidly beneath her eyelids as she slept, and she suddenly let out an anguished and haunting moan that scared the bejesus out of me. I wondered what demons she was battling in that head of hers.

I gently stroked her hair. Well, I stroked what was left of it. Her hair had been coming out in clumps the last few days and now was really patchy. She'd been wearing a worn-in Tulane hat by day, so this was the first close, long look I'd gotten. It was heartbreaking. The shiny thick hair that normally went down to the middle of her back was now less than shoulder length. That was just what was left. The remainder was in clumps, most of it gone in front, leaving Cali looking like a man with a receding hairline who refused to go to the barber to clean up the patches. The sides were going now too, which I hadn't previously noticed. There really were only a few wisps of hair left, which looked fine coming out from under a hat but was really knocking me for a loop now, with her pale scalp shining through.

She also looked beautiful. I'd felt this way when she had our babies too. Giving birth must be the least glamorous time for a woman.

Being in pain, discomfort, pushing, fighting, sweating, crying, and cursing do not equate to what I'd say is traditionally sexy. But I fell more in love with Cali back then, and this situation was having the same effect. Cali was a warrior, lying down to rest momentarily as she prepared for another day of battle. In that moment, I was so proud to be her husband.

CHAPTER 22
Digging a Hole

I'm standing at the second entrance to our neighborhood. Before the houses begin, the first few hundred feet of the road are bordered by several acres of wooded valley on each side. Since there are no leaves yet, I can see deep into the woods.

I am doing work on The Woodlands entrance. Maybe I am planting something or fixing a sign or a light. It is not clear, but I am focused. I glance up just in time to see a pack of wolves sneaking up on me from the valley. They are spread out, forming a deep inverted V shape that extends back down into the woods. The wolves on the flanks are closer. As I look up, they freeze, midstep, their eyes glowing eerily. The nearest wolf is on my left, a white-and-gray alpha, standing alert with one paw up. He slowly places his hoof (or paw) to the ground and bares his sharp yellow teeth, emitting a low, horrible growl from deep in his throat.

I look down and see I am holding the original survey of my property. I recently located this document for the pool guys, and it was like striking gold. Finding it was pure luck, and it saved me a few bucks since it didn't have to be redone. Since then, I've been keeping it front and center on my desk, the valuable blueprint folded up into a large thick rectangle.

It is the only tool I have with which to defend myself, so I bend slightly and slap the folded document against the asphalt road, making a loud popping sound. The lead wolf takes a step back. I whack the ground again and notice the rest of *the pack is hesitant now as well. I continue slapping the folded survey against the road. Each time I do this, though, the thick document deteriorates more and more. Eventually, it is just a handful of shredded paper. Although the wolves begin their creeping approach anew, all I can focus on now is that I've destroyed this valuable document.*

Finally, I lower my head and let out my own guttural, low growl, puffing up my (already puffy) body and taking a step forward. The wolves back off, slowly and reluctantly retreating into the woods.

The dream ended there, but I woke up feeling that the threat was not gone. Not completely. Maybe not ever. I lay there for a minute. I love interpreting dreams and couldn't help but wonder: Was I throwing this pool at Cali's cancer as a bandage and destroying our finances in the process?

★ ★ ★

Ed the Engineer came over to take a look around so he could eventually draw up plans for said pool. Ed was an older gentleman referred by the pool company. He stood waiting for me beside his old pickup truck, which was leaking oil onto my driveway. He had no mask on. I made a flamboyant show of putting mine on as I left the house, but Ed didn't take the hint. I explained that even though I'd been vaccinated, I was being extra careful by wearing the mask because my wife had a compromised immune system. He gave a nod, approving my caution. He didn't mask up though.

I let it go because he was an old-timer who probably didn't believe in germs, or science, and I didn't want to get off on the wrong foot with the guy who could railroad this whole project if he got his undies in a bunch. Politics and differences in personal beliefs seem to create problems now more than ever.

We walked the property. I say *property* like it's some sprawling estate. It's a normal house lot. Front and back yards. Ed didn't take notes. He didn't say much. He walked so slowly that I often stopped, wondering if he was following me or not. When we concluded our tour, Ed then informed me of roughly ten things that could prevent us from installing a pool, including the fact that we were surrounded by wetlands, which are environmentally protected. My butthole tightened.

We moseyed back around to his car, where I wrote Ed a check for a ridiculous amount, considering he basically had to draw a little pool onto my existing property survey and file some paperwork. I could have done it in crayon right there for twenty-six cents. Then he pulled out another document I had to sign, authorizing that the town could come do a wetlands survey. I wrote another check, this time to the town of Somers.

As he shoehorned himself into his truck, I asked Ed how long the process would take.

He finished settling in with the door ajar and said, "If the town does the wetlands survey and approves the application, you'll have permits within a month. If not, you have to go in front of the town board, and you're losing the summer. Plus, that ain't included in my fee."

He drove off, slowly. No rush.

CHAPTER 23
Playdate

My boss Mitchell called me. I could hear traffic and city noises, along with his heavier breathing, which all led me to deduce he was walking the city streets. Mitchell was fired up about how the world was getting back to normal, and the stores and events and markets were opening up, and it would have a positive impact on sales, and it was time for the world to get back to work, and if I wanted to come into the city sometime soon for lunch, we could catch up in person, and also he was heading down to Miami for the week, and then the following week he would be in Virginia, visiting our factory, but after that, his schedule was wide open if I wanted to get together.

I hung up the phone, frazzled. It was April 8, 2021.

I thought about driving into the city again. That disgusting commute had nearly killed me and crushed my soul. I pictured parking in a lot and having some random dude in my car, touching everything. I imagined myself walking the city streets, surrounded by people. Many of whom, based on percentages, would completely ignore the mask and distance guidelines, walking closely to me, breathing on me, brushing against me. I envisioned the filth and muck with which I would surely come into contact on the subway when I gripped that metal pole in the center of the train. Or riding in a taxi, which was a petri dish on wheels. I thought about getting on an elevator and sharing that small space with others, imagining a little incubation chamber that moved floor to floor, slowly cultivating germs. And I then imagined seeing Mitchell and somehow refraining from hugging him—we are big huggers. And finally, I imagined bringing all those germs back to an uninoculated Cali with her compromised immune system, like a big, gift-wrapped turd.

Then I thought about going back to doing that every day. That got me woozy. The sense of dread and fear was overwhelming. How the hell was I going to handle a return to normalcy?

Yes, I had gotten both Pfizer vaccines. I drove down to the Westchester County Center just last week to get my other shot. The whole experience was way less interesting the second time around, although the scene hadn't changed and still had the same, crazy postapocalyptic vibe. Funny what you can get used to, or scary what you can get used to ….

Also funny, that same day I got a ticket in the mail from when I'd driven into White Plains for my first vaccine. I remember being a little disoriented with all the road closures and rerouting as I weaved toward the parking area. Apparently, I went through a red light. Caught by a robotic camera.

Robots! I shook my fist in the air, like when William Shatner yelled, "Kahn!" in the second *Star Trek* movie.

Anyway, while I hoped everyone would be vaccinated soon, it had just come out that the J&J vaccine was causing blood clots, and they were pulling it. Pfizer had announced that people would need booster shots, which meant it wears off, which meant everyone's would wear off at different times. There also were other strains that might not be covered by the current vaccines. And, while the vaccine helped prevent people from getting COVID, there was no scientific proof that it prevented you from carrying it and giving it to someone else. It felt like the pandemic was never going to be over.

Plus, I liked my current situation. I didn't have to wake up as early anymore. Didn't have to shower as often; gross but true. I was getting tons of work done, but if I wanted to take a break, I could walk right into my kitchen for a snack or step out on the deck for some air. I was more likely to check emails in the evening because I wasn't completely toasted from a day circumnavigating the city and driving in and out of traffic. I had begun drawing and painting again over the last year. I was more present, more creative, more alive. I no longer struggled to sleep at night, dreading the next morning's drive, nor did I spend the entire Sunday in a miserable mood anticipating the vehicular tortures that lay ahead of me. I listened to the news less since I wasn't in the car, which was a good thing because the news had almost made my head explode over the previous four years. I was eventually going to use the extra time to exercise on a regular basis. It had only been a year; I was working up to it.

During hunting season, I was occasionally able to get in the woods before sunrise, hunt for three hours, and come back in by 9 a.m. for a full day of work. And now that spring had sprung, I could do the same with fishing. I keep a rowboat on the Croton Falls Reservoir nearby. I'm embarrassed to say I haven't used it in three years. It would be nice to get back into that.

Most importantly, this new freedom allowed me to be present for Cali.

I knew I was lucky to have a job. And I was grateful. But I'd had a taste of a better quality of life and been just as, if not more, productive. I didn't want to let that go.

★ ★ ★

I told you Cali and I are cautiously social. We don't want to get sucked into a suffocating relationship; therefore, we don't enter many new relationships. There was this one couple, Tracy and Glenn, whom we'd been circling around a little though, and they had showed genuine concern about Cali when they heard the news.

We knew Tracy and Glenn because they were friends with everyone but us. We'd seen them at parties, mostly. I could tell Tracy was cool right out of the gate—super friendly and talkative with no air of snobbery. She just reminded me of a good-old Long Island girl, which, it turned out, she was.

Her husband Glenn gave a different first, and second, impression. I'm not afraid to say it: Glenn is rather handsome. He's in great shape, has dark hair and blue eyes, and always has that exact-same-length five-o'clock shadow. How do guys maintain that? My beard is generally a multi-length disaster.

Glenn also has a quiet demeanor I initially mistook for arrogance.

So, if we were out and their names came up, I'd ask, "How is that guy?" Half-expecting to get some dirt and justify my suspicions.

Every time, no dirt.

"He's a solid dude."

"He's a really good guy."

Ugh.

I wanted to dislike this guy, but no one was letting me.

Then we wound up having dinner with him and Tracy. We had plans with our friends Dan and Amy, and at the last minute Amy texted to see if it was okay for them to join us. Cali gave her approval. I immediately wanted to cancel, imagining Dan and Glenn, who have been friends for a while, talking about their last round of golf or their kids' lacrosse game or anything else that would exclude me from participating.

Anyway, dinner was nice, and Glenn was nice. It was all nice.

That was a few months back. I hadn't seen or spoken to Glenn since. Then few days ago, he'd sent me a text saying he was sorry to hear about Cali, and if there was anything he could do to help, I should just let him know.

I imagined his wife coercing him to send that text, and Glenn doing so begrudgingly, muttering that he barely knows me. But really, that was *me* I was imagining.

And if you need to vent or just get out and grab a drink, I'm there, he added.

Okay, sounds good, I typed, acknowledging what I perceived as the obligatory empty offer.

That's what friends are for, he responded.

"That's what friends are for" was not really one of those compulsory responses. Maybe Glenn was the real deal. No one is so shady, they would add that last line if they didn't mean it. In fact, it seemed he was going out of his way to make it clear he meant it.

I tend to overthink things.

That morning, I got a follow-up text from Glenn, saying he'd be done with work at 4:30 p.m. and asking if I wanted to go grab that drink. I stared at my phone for a while, already feeling the awkwardness of a one-on-one with someone I barely knew. My instinct was to make up an excuse and bow out while expressing my gratitude. My thumbs hovered over my phone's virtual keyboard, about to work their magic. *Keep Gregg safe from outside agitators, thumbs. Keep Gregg in his comfort zone, thumbs.*

My thumbs had a different idea. My thumbs knew I was having an awakening of sorts, and this was important. My goddamn thumbs typed, Sounds great! See you later.

Of course, it turned out totally fine with Glenn. I met him at an outside table at a local joint. The weather was perfect, and we sat there in the setting sun, drinking beers and talking about everything two guys getting to know each other might cover.

The conversation continued, and the waiter kept bringing more beers for some strange reason. Eventually, we were both buzzed and hungry, so we ordered a couple of burgers. I texted Cali to go ahead and eat without me.

She wrote back, Ooh your date must be going well!

Glenn didn't share his political opinions, and I didn't either. He didn't talk sports too much, and we still managed to have an easy conversation that never got awkward or uncomfortable. At one point, I mentioned Cali, and he asked about her in a very careful way as if to say, *You can get into this or not. It's up to you.*

So I got into it a little. He listened. I didn't want to bore him to death, but it was helpful for me to talk about these things with someone. Hours later, we bumped fists in the parking lot, the air growing a little colder now that the sun was low. We agreed to do it again some time.

CHAPTER 24
Market Driver

The week of April 15, 2021 was somewhat uneventful, which was a good thing. Cali was feeling fine but very tired. She would do a few things around the house and then collapse either on the couch or upstairs in bed. Then she would watch *Law & Order*.

Cali is addicted to that show. There must be one channel that only plays *Law & Order* because it is always on. And there are multiple versions, *Law & Order: Special Victims Unit*, *Law & Order: Criminal Intent*, etc. Now there's one about organized crime. I'm expecting more spin-offs.

Law & Order: Shoplifting.

Law & Order: Public Urination.

Each time an episode ends, another one starts right up. They don't even take a commercial break, so Cali gets pulled right in. This is when she exclaims, "I saw this one! It's so good," or "Oh my God! I never saw this one somehow." It doesn't matter. Either way, she'll watch.

I believe there is a subliminal track running in the background of that show that hypnotizes the viewer. If I happen to walk into the room when it is on, I find myself standing there minutes later, watching, slack-jawed. "Wait. He killed his twin brother? The DJ?"

Cali gets so excited when I get sucked in.

Cali also watches the *Housewives* shows on Bravo. Those are just a hot mess with everyone shouting at each other, and it's incredibly stupid and puts out such terrible energy that I can't believe anyone would ... "Wait. She slept with her best friend's brother? The one in *jail*?"

Garbage. But I get drawn into those shows too.

As *Law & Order* played, our phone rang. Our landline always announces the caller ID, and it was normally Cali's mom or sister in the evening. Several times that week, the phone rang and announced an unusual number. Cali paced around the kitchen and dining room while talking, but I could overhear.

"Oh, thank you. Yes, it will be a few more months. That's so sweet. No, I miss you too."

This happened a few nights in a row, so I finally asked who the hell was calling. Turns out, they really missed her at the hair salon, the nail place, Bloomingdale's, and everywhere else that was going out of business since my wife wasn't there every day. Cali being homebound was impacting entire industries.

CHAPTER 25
Psychic Love Connection

That Saturday morning, April 17, 2021, was sunny and looking to be a warm one. We were eating breakfast, and I was looking forward to a day of nothing. Cali's phone dinged. Cali read the text, typed back, and then announced that Brenda and Michael were stopping by. We would sit on the deck with them. This was a big progression from the front steps, where we normally welcomed them. The deck seemed more official than a casual stopover. I had serious plans to ignore my to-do list all day, so this was a huge inconvenience.

But New Gregg enjoyed people. New Gregg appreciated anyone who went out of their way for us. New Gregg was breaking out of his comfort zone and expanding his horizons. New Gregg would benefit from this by having a fuller and more connected life. Not that New Gregg had a choice in this particular instance.

Of course, it turned out to be enjoyable. Brenda and Michael spent just the right amount of time out there on the deck with us. We chatted casually, and they knew exactly when to leave. Maybe because after an hour, I stood up from the table and pushed my chair in, but at least they took the hint.

That was perfect. Cali was pleased, I had fulfilled my social duties for the day, and it was only 1 p.m. I had the rest of the day to not do anything I was supposed to.

A few minutes later, Cali looked at her phone. "Aaron and Shari are going to come over after Hayden's game. They'll probably stay for dinner."

Her phone hated me.

I was going to smash it and finally be free.

Distressed, I rambled, "What time are they coming? We don't even know what time? What am I supposed to do until then if I don't even know when they are coming? What are we doing with them? Just hanging out? Are they staying for dinner? What time are they leaving? I'm tired already from Brenda and Michael. I have nothing left in the tank. Why? Why are we doing this? Couldn't we have discussed it? Are your parents coming too?"

I was a huge cranky jerk for the next few hours. Anything Cali said, I brought it back to how miserable I was and how my *whole weekend* had been ruined.

Cali was initially apologetic but began to grow irritated and then angry. "Will you stop being such a baby? I want to see my sister."

Right. Once again, I had forgotten this was not all about me. I could suck it up for Cali. Plus, I enjoy hanging out with Shari and Aaron. I don't know why I get like that.

They came over later that afternoon. Aaron and I went down to the basement and sat at the bar, making different cocktails and then, you know, drinking them. We ordered dinner. Afterward, Aaron and I went back down to the bar and made more cocktails. And drank them. Down there in the basement, Aaron and I had a long, deep conversation. We discussed Cali's illness and Aaron's late mother Georgie, who'd had lymphoma. How I was feeling, *really* feeling about things. We talked about the kids, our jobs, what things would be like after COVID. If there *were* an after. We got drunk. Then we got more drunk. I didn't check my watch, and I didn't wonder when they were leaving.

When we came upstairs, I heard something that warmed my drunken heart. Cali was laughing. Laughing *hysterically*. Cali and Shari were sitting on the couch, looking at Cali's phone. They were watching TikTok videos; just stupid thirty-second clips of people dancing or getting kicked in the nuts or mauled by an animal. But they were both laughing so hard, with tears streaming down their faces.

It was so great to see. Cali really needed that. Maybe I did too. It was a good night.

★ ★ ★

Cali and I have a Sunday morning routine. I go out and get the newspapers. Cali stands at the counter reading and eating a cup of dry cereal or something, and I sit at the table and eat like a normal human. I attempt to read the paper, but Cali calls out anything she finds interesting in her section, which is everything. This happens every thirty seconds or so. I read the same headline forty times or just blast through the paper without comprehending anything since Cali is essentially reading me her section of the paper. It would be like turning on CNN and Fox News at the same time, but while you were trying to relax and eat.

It used to infuriate me, but now I kind of like it. I've been appreciating Cali's little quirks more and more lately; I suppose since I often think about what life would be like without them.

Anyway, it was rare, but Cali had beaten me downstairs and was standing at the kitchen island in her PJs and reading the Sunday paper when I walked into the room. It was still shocking to see how small she looked, and how much hair she had lost. She was scheduled to begin her third round of chemo the next day. I knew she must be nervous, and I suddenly felt the desire to comfort her.

I took her by the arms and turned her away from the newspaper. I put my hands up to cradle her face and gently angled it up so I could look deeply into her eyes. I just wanted to connect with her on a different level, to soothe her for a moment without all the outside noise of newspapers, television, and text messages. I opened my mouth to tell her I would be there for her no matter what, that I knew she was nervous but wanted her to know she was not alone.

She spoke first. "The sprinkler guys are coming next weekend to turn the outside water back on."

Okay, fair enough. I hadn't made my intentions clear. "Forget about the sprinklers, Cali. Let's just take a moment before you start round three tomorrow to connect. I just want to look into your eyes and shut everything else out, so you feel supported."

She nodded.

I began the magical psychic love connection process I had just invented.

Cali spoke. "They raised the price of the *Journal News* again. I'm calling them and threatening to cancel."

Argh! This was going to be impossible.

Cali pulled away from me and turned back to the paper. "Also, can you change the lightbulb in our bathroom over the tub? I know you just changed it, but it seems dimmer than the others."

I gave up and looked at Cali's tiny head, laughing to myself. *It must be noisy in there.*

CHAPTER 26
Round Three

Tuesday, April 20, 2021, was Cali's second day of round three. I was feeling frustrated. It felt like we'd been doing this forever, and we weren't even halfway through. After these three weeks, it would officially be halfway. The doctor said they were going to do a PET scan after this round to see if everything was working, so I was anxiously eager to get to that.

I woke up early and drove Ella to school. They had reopened the school to everyone, so there were no more staggered groups of people at home. No one was willing to ride the bus, though, so there was a major traffic jam starting half a mile away from the school. Ella couldn't drive herself yet, and juniors were not allowed to park at the school anyway. Some of her friends drove and parked at some kid's house nearby, but I was not making Ella walk almost a mile each morning, crossing major roads, with her giant backpack of schoolbooks, her lacrosse stick, and her other huge backpack filled with lacrosse gear.

Ella was nervous during the drive. Her second round of lacrosse tryouts were that afternoon, so I tried to loosen her up a bit. I cranked up the radio and started doing the robot while steering with my knee.

Are you not entertained!?

I got home just in time to drive Cali to chemo. Traffic was heavier than usual. More people were venturing out. It was stressing me out. I dropped Cali off at the hospital and drove back home. One hour round trip.

I finally sat down and started to work when the smart doorbell told me there was someone at the door. I was glad I looked because it was the town wetlands inspector, showing up unannounced. I couldn't blow him off because one small delay could completely derail our pool plans, so I took him for a walk around the backyard. A half hour later, he had thoroughly inspected my wetlands to his satisfaction, which sounds dirty but is not.

I went inside to dive into some work emails. Ella had a short school day, though, so I soon left again to pick her up. Her schedule didn't line up with any of her friends' schedules, and she had no ride home.

I arrived home with Ella just in time to leave the house again. I had to pick Cali up at 1 p.m. When I arrived, Cali was very tired but otherwise okay. She slumped into the car and dozed a bit on the way home. One hour round trip.

I got home in time to leave *again* so I could drive Ella to lacrosse tryouts at the school. At that point, I decided to just wait at the school for her practice/tryouts to be over an hour and a half later. I simply didn't want to drive home and back again. So I sat in my car, although I was so tempted to disguise myself as a bush and sit near the field to spy on her tryouts.

The good news, aside from Cali feeling okay, was that the wetlands inspector didn't anticipate any issues.

And Ella made varsity.

We thought.

Halfway through tryouts, the coach split the group of girls in two. Ella was with all seniors and a handful of underclassmen who were clearly the stronger players. The other group went off with the JV coach. Ella's group stayed with the varsity coaches.

The coach said, "Okay, let's swing the ball around a little. Get used to the people around you. You're gonna be playing with them this season."

Ella relayed this story to us, and Cali and I said almost simultaneously, "Congratulations! You made varsity!"

Ella said, "No. They didn't officially announce it."

So even though we wanted to tell everyone, Ella wouldn't let us because it wasn't official. I got it. She didn't want to jinx anything. Enough had gone wrong for her recently.

★ ★ ★

On Wednesday morning, I woke and stared at the ceiling, gathering my strength for another day. I rolled over to check on Cali. That's the first thing I did lately; just to make sure everything was okay over there on her side of the bed.

Cali opened her eyes. As if she could read my struggling mind, she immediately told me how much she appreciated everything I'd been doing. I needed that. It made the day instantly more endurable. After a frustrating day of driving all over the place yesterday, I wasn't totally looking forward to today, even though Cali only had a short session.

Ella came home from school that day and announced it was official. She'd made varsity. In reality, it wasn't any more official today than it had been yesterday, but when she asked a few girls if these were the teams, they all said, "Yes, what is wrong with you?"

Hunter texted me from Columbus to say he'd been rejected from two of seven internships to which he'd applied.

I encouraged him to widen the net a bit and apply to more. Seven wasn't going to do the trick.

He wrote, *We'll see.*

That night, Cali suddenly jumped up and ran to the bathroom to take her anti-nausea medication. It helped, but she felt strange all night.

CHAPTER 27
Venturing Out

That Friday, everything hit Cali hard. She felt awful and stayed in bed all day, asleep to the soothing sounds of *Law & Order*. This was the worst I had seen her. She couldn't move and didn't want to. I could tell it was bad because she wasn't even apologizing for feeling lousy. Normally, she apologized at least ten times a day for no reason. As if she'd gotten sick on purpose, and we were all mad about it. I kept begging her to stop apologizing all the time.

We'd be eating and Cali, with tears welling up in her eyes, would say to me and Ella, "I'm sorry I'm sick."

We would stop eating and say, "What? Don't apologize. We love you. We are happy to be here for you. Just stop it, that's silly."

An hour later, the tears would come back, and Cali would say, "I just feel like I'm not pulling my weight. I feel terrible that we've ordered dinner the last three nights. I couldn't even do the laundry today. I really am sorry."

And we would say, "Are you crazy? You shouldn't be doing those things anyway. You should be letting us do them, but you won't. Now stop apologizing and focus on healing. That's all you should be thinking about."

Later, she'd be crying again and say, "It's my job to do all these things, and I'm letting you all down. I feel terrible. I'm so sorry."

At this point, I'd be done. "Cali, when you apologize, it makes it seem like I'm actually upset about this. Which I am not. So I'm sitting here, accepting your apology, as if I were really pissed and now, I'm saying, 'Hey, it's okay.' And now, this *is* irritating me. So, *stop apologizing.*"

Cali would sulk after this and, now irritated herself, would say sarcastically, "*Sorry.*"

★★★

Cali still felt rotten on Monday morning after a difficult weekend, but in the afternoon, she announced she was going with me to Ella's first lacrosse game. Cali hadn't really been out in public, aside from her doctor appointments. I told her she didn't have to go. Ella would understand, and I'd be there representing. She insisted.

The game was great. I'd missed this. Hunter and Alix had both run track, and Alix also played high school soccer. Her soccer team was amazing, and the team competed at a high level, which was very exciting. I never missed an event and took great pleasure watching them compete. I would often drive home early from the city to catch a game, changing out of my suit in the car while driving. Which wasn't that difficult since I was normally stuck in traffic, creeping along at two miles per hour.

Ella had played lacrosse the last few years in a rec league. Then she played on JV during her freshman year of high school, but COVID stole her sophomore season like it had so many other things.

It was just nice to be at an event. People were really getting vaccinated now, and although the school was strict about only allowing two guests per player, enforcing the mask mandate, and trying to keep people six feet apart with markers on the stands, it was just perfect to be around people again.

I can't believe I just said that.

In fact, guess who showed up to Ella's first game? That's right. New Gregg. Yes, New Gregg climbed up those stands with Cali in tow and proceeded to introduce himself to anyone he didn't recognize. I probably already knew half of them and just forgot, which might have explained some of the strange looks. We were going to be spending some time together, with our daughters being on the same team, and I thought it was important to get to know everyone. I knew some of the other parents already from lacrosse or just around town, but I made a point to greet everyone.

Cali stared at me the whole time. "Who *are* you?"

It was a little weird though. Cali didn't exactly have a sign on her that said, "I have cancer," but I wondered.

To someone who hadn't seen her in over a year due to COVID, was it obvious she was forty-five pounds lighter?

Would they wonder why she was wearing a bandana on her head, or was that a fashionable thing people wear now?

Would they notice the little wisps of hair flowing out the back? That she was walking funny, looked weak, seemed sick?

And did I look fat?

CHAPTER 28
Wake-Up Call

At the end of March, I had visited my doctor for a routine blood test. A week later, his receptionist called me. She read through the results at breakneck speed, and although I attempted to take notes, I was missing half of what she said. Normally, the doctor would take me through this information, and I could ask, "Is that bad? Is that bad?" There was no dialogue this time.

As she read, the receptionist commented, "Ooh, I think that's high. Oh, that's not a great number."

Then she said that due to the results, the doctor really felt it was time for me to make some life changes. She did not specify what those changes were. And while logic could dictate what they might be, I didn't want to make assumptions. Maybe I was supposed to eat *more* pizza and ice cream. You never know.

She also said the doctor wanted to get me on a specific drug, for which it was very difficult to get the insurance companies to agree to pay, so he wanted me to go for an ultrasound of my carotid artery. If they found buildup or anything else lodged in there, he could prescribe this medication and insurance would cover it. He would call in the ultrasound order to Northeast Radiology in Mt. Kisco.

Then I pretended that conversation never happened and did nothing for two weeks.

Two weeks later, I received a phone call. We answer calls now, whereas in the past we ignored them. We technically do not even need a landline in our house. We all have cell phones and only have a landline to screen calls from solicitors and so Cali can talk to her mom on not a cell phone. Nowadays, it could be something important and medically related to Cali, so I picked up the phone when I saw Northeast Radiology on the caller ID.

The woman asked for Gregg Goldman, though, and seemed perplexed when I didn't immediately know why she was calling. They'd had an order for a carotid ultrasound there for two weeks, but I never made an appointment. This is normally an urgent procedure, and the patient wants to get in there right away.

Oops.

I made an appointment for April 14.

When that day arrived, I headed over to Northeast Radiology and they eventually escorted me to a room toward the back of the building. Per the technician's instructions, I stripped down to my underwear, got under a sheet, and waited for her to come back in. The tech then slathered blue goo on a wand and began sliding it around the right side of my neck, I assume recording various angles of my artery. I was familiar with an ultrasound from Cali's pregnancies, but I certainly would have freaked out if the screen showed a baby in my neck. The technician explained that this carotid exam would take forty-five minutes and then she would do the same to my groin/leg area. That would take an hour. She examined the carotid artery, clicking away on the keyboard, taking measurements of length, diameter, and, most importantly, girth. She was looking for a blockage, obstruction, or anything else that might look strange, perhaps a hunk of steak or an old cigarette butt.

I used the time to do absolutely nothing. I couldn't look at my phone or talk to the tech because it would screw up the results. I hovered there in a half-asleep dreamlike state, thinking about Cali. Then I thought about the kids, and work, and various other things. When she got down to my groinal area, I thought about baseball.

Part of me wanted them to find something. I know that sounds insane, but it would explain a lot. I know I am out of shape and overweight, but I feel disproportionately lethargic and sluggish. If I exert myself just a bit, I easily get lightheaded and dizzy. If I sit up after lying down, I get the spins and see stars. If I tilt my head back, everything spins. Simple yard work I used to be able to do for hours is now parsed out over a few hundred weekends because I've only got twenty minutes before I am covered in sweat and it feels like all the blood has drained from my head and body.

I know I've ridden this horse hard for many of my forty-eight years, but I know other people who did the same, and they don't get worn out so easily. So, yes, part of me was hoping they'd find something. It would suck, but it would finally explain things. I would deal with whatever had to be done and, hopefully, have an improved quality of life afterward. It was bad timing with Cali, but it would be a relief, in a way.

A week later, the doctor's receptionist called. She was speed-reading the notes again, and it certainly was not akin to Morgan Freeman narrating a documentary about the mating habits of penguins. In fact, it wasn't even as clear as a New York City subway announcement. I spaced out immediately, angry and distracted that my doctor didn't call me personally. I did gather that they found nothing from the ultrasound, which was good news, I suppose. Yet, they found just enough of *something* to get the insurance company to agree to the medication, which was also good news. What they found and the medication she was talking about was still a mystery, even though she probably told me.

A few days later, I'd been making my weekly pilgrimage to the Stop & Shop Pharmacy to pick up Cali's meds when the pharmacist realized he had something for me too. We were all cool now, me and the rogue gang of roughneck pharmacists. He went to the refrigerator, which is where they keep the good shit, and took out four boxes. He bagged the boxes and stapled on a long, multipage instructional document.

I scanned the documentation when I got home, noticing there was a section about how to administer the injection to yourself, and an even longer section about the possible side effects. No one had said anything about injections. Enough was enough. I called the office and said I wanted to speak with the doctor.

When I got on the Zoom call on Wednesday, April 28, with Dr. G., I was ready to complain like a lady named Barb at a South Carolina Chick-fil-A. But the doc is so nice and gentle that he defused me quickly, and I just let it go. I realized I was really angry because I had let myself go so badly and not just that the doctor hadn't called me personally.

Bottom line was, my blood sugar and cholesterol and insulin and glucose and a few other things were all too high, despite all the meds I was already on. Rather than increase the statin I was taking for cholesterol, which could have significant side effects and limited results, the doc wanted to get me on this other medication. It is expensive though, and he needed to do that ultrasound thing to get me approved.

They found nothing major in the ultrasound but just enough plaque, which mostly everyone has anyway, to justify the medication. The medication was an injection I gave myself once every two weeks and would help greatly. That was it.

I then asked what he meant by "time to make some changes," which the receptionist had managed to convey, and it disappointingly turned out to be what I'd expected. I had to really make changes to my diet and make exercise part of my daily routine. I eagerly listened to his suggestions, intending to get started as soon as we hung up. It was time.

We hung up. I didn't do anything.

I had Taco Bell for dinner that night, I shit you not.

CHAPTER 29

An Attention-Starved, Insecure,
ADD-Riddled Infant

Another weekend, another visit from Cali's parents. Overlapping with and followed by a visit from Shari and Aaron that lasted well into the night.

Cali's parents came over around 2 p.m. I normally would have made myself scarce, but I had already vanished the last few times they visited. I knew they were there to visit their sick daughter and not me, but I figured it might be rude if I didn't stick around occasionally.

The weather was nice, so we sat outside on the deck. No one said a word to me the entire time as they chatted about this and that. I made a little joke at one point. No one laughed. I got bored.

Then Big Al focused his attention on me and offered me some advice. "You need more color out front in the landscaping. It looks terrible. You ever see my house? I have lots of color. I planted them all myself. You got no color."

I steamed, silently. That very week, I had spent over $1,000 on new plants and bushes, moved some existing ones around, and put down fresh mulch in all the beds. It looked beautiful out there. I excused myself and went inside, turning on the very early Kentucky Derby coverage and mixing myself an Old Fashioned to get in the spirit. I didn't go back out.

Around 6 p.m., Shari and Aaron arrived. Cali's parents left after seeing them for a while.

Aaron and I had a few bourbons in honor of the Kentucky Derby, a nice bottle of wine with dinner, then a few scotches afterward in honor of overdrinking. By 10:30 p.m., I was drunk and full, nursing a dull headache, and had zero energy. Also, my ADD meds had worn off, and I was done for the night.

Shari had fallen asleep sitting up on the couch, phone in hand. Aaron found a movie he had already seen fourteen times and turned it on halfway through. At the same time, Cali got an alert confirming our food order on DoorDash, which was strange because we hadn't ordered anything. Then she got an alert from a different restaurant. And finally, a third. We quickly deduced that someone had hacked our DoorDash account and ordered three separate meals for pickup at three separate restaurants in Brooklyn. While Cali was frantically on the phone with the bank, trying to put a hold on the card associated with our account, I was trying to reach DoorDash to cancel the orders and let them know what was happening. I secretly wished the fuckers who'd hacked us had ordered delivery instead of pickup because I was drunk and angry enough to show up to their address with my Louisville Slugger.

In his defense, Aaron was also drunk but seemingly oblivious to what we were dealing with because he had the movie volume cranked up loud. He kept talking to us about the movie, even though we were both frantic on the phone, clearly not watching the movie, and not responding to him in any way. I was getting more and more irritated. When we had finally resolved as much as we could with the DoorDash thing late in the evening, I let out a sigh of relief and looked at Aaron knowingly, expecting him to turn off the movie, wake up his wife, and say it was time to go.

He did not.

I looked at Cali, sending her a psychic message with my widened eyes. She received my signal and announced she was tired and had to go to sleep. Shari and Aaron made their way to the door. I was halfway upstairs with my shirt off before they even got to their car.

Cali came up and started getting ready for bed. "That was nice," she said.

"Oh, was it?" I asked.

"What's wrong?"

"Oh, nothing!" I said sarcastically. "It was so nice spending my *entire Saturday* with your family. Nothing I'd rather do after a week of hard work and driving you around than being ignored by your parents, having my landscaping insulted, and then having Shari and Aaron practically *move in*. It was a *fucking blast!*" My voice had grown louder. Some cultures might call it a yell.

Cali looked at me, washing off her makeup in the sink, her face dripping. "You're a dick," she observed. Rightfully so.

Cali was going through hell and just had had a wonderful visit with her parents and a nice and easy hang with her sister. This was all probably very comforting to her. Aside from the DoorDash situation, I could have had a nice time, too, if I weren't such an attention-starved, insecure, ADD-riddled infant.

Once again, I immediately felt terrible. I had to start catching these things *before* I screwed up and opened my mouth. I apologized, sincerely. My apology was not totally accepted.

We went to bed.

CHAPTER 30
Tensions Are Rising

On Wednesday, May 5, Hunter—having concluded his junior year—came home from Ohio State. He'd driven home with a kid from his fraternity who lived nearby. They hit some traffic from an accident in Pennsylvania and lost an hour, so he got in a little later than planned. Overall, it took around ten hours door-to-door. Not terrible.

I met him in the driveway, and we hugged. Hunter is six feet tall, just like me, but is maybe a half inch taller than me. I helped him unload his bags from the Jeep into the front hallway. He had packed frantically and moved out of the fraternity house in the last two days because he'd been busy with finals and papers up until then. All his furniture went into storage in Columbus; his clothing was stuffed into blue IKEA bags, which he brought home.

Over Christmas break, Hunter had been home for over a month and never unpacked his clothing. He just lived out of a few bags he left open on his floor. This drove me bonkers, and I did not want that to happen this summer. Hunter had also stayed up until 4 a.m. and slept until 2 p.m. over the last break, which I suspected was his normal schedule back at school too. I was not cool with that either and hoped that would change this summer as well. He'd presumably have an internship or a job, so that would get him out of bed, although, again, he should have booked an internship months ago.

Hunter told us he'd been feeling down that last week or two at school, which was difficult to imagine. Forget about his mom being sick; I got that. But he lived in a fraternity house with twenty-eight of his best buds. There was always something going on. They had parties on the weekend, parties during the day; sometimes a party broke out during a party. The weather had been getting nicer, and as Hunter had been knocking off one final after the other over the last few weeks, the COVID restrictions had been lifted too. He could've gone to the bars and really had a blast if he wanted.

Yet during that time, if I reached out via text or phone call before 2 p.m., there was no response, increasing my suspicions that he was spending the day in bed. In fact, he normally wouldn't answer me until around 4 p.m., but he'd say he'd been taking a test or studying for the last two hours. I'd ask if he had any plans that night, and he'd say he didn't know. He sounded melancholy and bummed out. He said he was really stressed. When he said that, I immediately imagined he was stressed because he put off a project that was due the next day, which he should have been working on over the past three months. Or he was cramming for a test because he missed class and had to get the notes from someone. Maybe I was projecting since that was exactly what I'd done in college … if I even did that much.

His appearance had taken an interesting turn too. Hunter was a very handsome boy and had become a very handsome man. When he ran track in high school, his body had been totally ripped, and he had a real Danny Zuko look in that tracksuit. His fit physique clung to him those first two years of college, even though he no longer exercised or ran or lifted weights or walked. He had strong thumbs from playing video games, I'll give him that. This year, though, we could see on video calls—when his lights were on—that he was thin and pale. His hair was wild and longer than it had ever been. He pulled it into a man-bun occasionally, but otherwise, it was all over the place. I'm not saying it didn't look cool, but he just looked different. I was worried he wasn't taking great care of himself is all.

Either way, his grades were good, so if he finished college strong, that was all that mattered. Right? Or do the ends *not* justify the means? Were there some things, like character, desire, energy, and hard work, that mattered more? Was Hunter in a well-deserved but fleeting funk? Or was he morphing into something worrisome and more permanent?

Cali and I had discussed this before he came home. Would we be strict about making Hunter get out of bed at a reasonable hour, or had he earned a break after getting great grades? Would we insist he find an internship or job, or were we going to give him a pass because COVID had handed him a shitty year and screwed up a lot of in-person opportunities? Would we get on his ass to eat better, take care of himself physically and hygienically, or give the kid his freedom to do whatever he wanted? He had the rest of his life to conform. Plus, being a January baby, he was twenty-one already and entitled to make his own decisions.

We also had other, deeper questions for ourselves as parents. Were we too soft if we let him do his thing, whatever that might be? Would we be doing him a disservice if we weren't strict? Would good parents insist on his conformity or choose compassion? Was there a middle ground? It was all so much more complicated because of Cali's sickness.

Cali and I had discussed this *ad nauseum*. We finally agreed to give Hunter five days of relaxation before we brought anything up. Just let him see his mom, adjust to that whole situation, and then take his pulse and ease into things.

Our plan lasted less than twenty-four hours.

The next day, I was working but having a hard time focusing. With each hour that passed, it occurred to me that Hunter still hadn't woken up and come downstairs. I figured he'd be eager to spend some time with his mom, all things considered. Then again, he'd just had a crazy two weeks of finals and projects on top of stressing about his mom, saying "goodbye" to his friends, a frenzied two days of packing, and a long drive. I was sure he was beat and decided to give the kid another hour.

At 1 p.m., I angrily realized there was still no sign of Hunter. It didn't help I was having a wild day at work and, to my dismay, kept seeing Cali walk past my office with load after load of laundry. I told her to let me do it, but she was so stubborn. Hunter could have helped if he'd been up.

At 2 p.m., Hunter came down and made himself breakfast. Afterward, he popped his head into my office to say hello. I was so crabby by now, I could barely muster up any enthusiasm, even though it was still good to see him after all this time.

I held my tongue as we made small talk, and I remembered my pact with Cali to stay off his ass until Monday. But then he brought up his internship search and said he had a few things in mind he would work on. I supposed this meant he was okay with talking about these things, so I jumped in. I told him that his mom and I had agreed to wait until Monday, but since he'd mentioned it, we were going to tell him on Monday that he had a week to find an internship or would have to get an actual job. That he had to be unpacked within a week, unlike Christmas break. That since he'd had the Jeep at school all year, he was to take it to get washed and then serviced. That he needed to eat better and take better care of his hygiene. And hey, doesn't getting out of bed by 11 a.m. sound fair?

His face dropped. He said, "Okay," and walked out.

Later, I opened the door to the garage but immediately forgot why I was going in there, so I went back into my office. I had set off the open-door chime on our alarm system though, and Hunter must have thought I went out.

As I sat at my desk, I overheard him complaining about someone to Cali. He was pissed about some asshole who had jumped all over him and couldn't even leave him alone for a day. He didn't know what this guy wanted from him. It took me a second, but I soon suspected I was the asshole of whom he spoke.

I asked, "Hunter, are you talking about *me* in there?"

He came in, followed by Cali. He said that yes, he was talking about me. Didn't I know what kind of stress he'd been through? How hard it was to come home and see his mother like this? How he just needed a break? He began sobbing as he spoke.

I felt terrible. Then I grew angry. I yelled, my voice quickly breaking into sobs, "Don't *I* know what you've been through? Don't *I* know it? Yes, *I* fucking know it! I've been working my balls off to keep this family afloat! To keep you in school and in your frat house palace. To keep Alix in New Orleans! To keep my customers and bosses happy while the world is crumbling around us! Driving Ella and your mom everywhere and trying to help around here, all while watching the woman I love fall apart in front of my eyes! Yes, I *fucking* know it! *You're* the one that doesn't know *shit*!" I was now screaming and standing and pointing.

He shut up. I shut up. I was out of breath. Cali started talking, trying to calm us down and remind us we were both stressed out and emotional. We cooled off and half-heartedly hugged it out.

They both left my office, but not before Cali paused and shot me a look. "You said we'd wait until Monday."

CHAPTER 31
Halfway Point

Cali had her halfway-point PET scan that Friday, May 7, 2021. Naturally, she was nervous. She was worried they'd tell her things had gotten worse or hadn't improved. She had also gotten feedback from her last routine mammography and was worried about that. They'd seen something, but I was sure it was a lymph node or related to something they already knew about. I told her not to worry. The lymph nodes that had been protruding out of her skin were no longer doing so. The doctors were absolutely going to tell her the treatment was working.

Hunter was asleep, but I wasn't asking him to do anything anyway, not after yesterday's episode. I woke early and drove Ella to school. Then I came back in time to bring Cali to her PET scan. The PET scans were done at a different hospital, so it was a nice change of scenery and a lovely drive through the winding roads of Putnam County. As we drove, the blooming trees and serene reservoirs breezed by.

There are many reservoirs in northern Westchester and lower Putnam County, many of which provide drinking water to New York State. There are no power boats or motorized vehicles allowed, so it can really be beautiful and peaceful driving around the area. I had a permit to fish the reservoirs. Seeing all this splendor reminded me of my rowboat on Croton Falls Reservoir that I hadn't used for over three years, which drove me crazy to think about.

I had been planning to wait for Cali at the hospital during her scan, even though it would take over two hours. I didn't want to do the drive back and forth and figured I'd work from my car. But the day before, an important customer had called and said we had to have a meeting at 10 a.m. the next day about a project, so I revised my plan and dropped Cali off. Then I drove home for the meeting, and it was a good thing I did because, halfway there, I had a battle with my butthole to avoid crapping in my shorts. That would have been a very different situation if I were still waiting in the parking lot.

I made it home just in the nick of time and hit the bathroom with fervor. I finished thirty seconds before my 10 a.m. meeting.

As I was logging on, Cali texted me.

Got done early. Come and get me!

Oh boy.

It was 10 a.m. exactly.

Again, I thought about waking Hunter, but aside from the tension, there would be no time to even explain where he should go, have him get ready, and then drive there without making Cali wait. It was also probably a bad idea to have him handle my work meeting, although I considered it. So I jumped in the car, dialed into the Zoom meeting, and drove to the hospital.

I don't remember the meeting or the drive, which is not good, but I did pull up to Cali standing outside the second the call ended, so it worked out okay. Surely, someone would've let me know if the meeting hadn't gone well ….

***

Dr. Fire-crotch had been very pleased to tell Cali some good news, and it was not about his neat new boat. The PET scan showed that the treatment was working, and she was making very positive progress. That was a huge relief. Although, I had been wondering about something lately. They couldn't originally tell for sure if Cali *had* cancer from the PET scan. They needed to take out a lymph node and test it. So, how were they going to tell from a PET scan that she *didn't* have cancer?

Either way, we were now officially past the halfway point as Cali began her fourth cycle on Monday, May 10, 2021. They had the *R* down to a science now, so there were no more rigors, and the session only took a few hours.

In other good news, I was expecting the pool permit any day now. Last week, I had texted Engineer Ed, asking when to expect it, and he replied that it would be mid-May. If I was figuring this out correctly, May is thirty-one days. *Mid*, as an English prefix, means "half." Half of thirty-one days is fifteen (and a half). So, by May 15, which was this week, it would be mid-May, and I could reasonably expect the permit to be issued.

There was a problem related to the pool, though, which I learned about at lacrosse of all places. Ella, by now, had played several lacrosse games. Her team was great and had a 4–0 record right out of the gate. There were a number of girls on the team committed to play in college next year, some Division 1. I was just fired up that Ella had made varsity and was playing at all. The games had been blowouts so far. We'd hoped for blowouts because then Ella would get playing time. When the team was up 8–0 ten minutes into the first half, Ella would go in. She was playing a full twenty minutes the first half and almost the entire second half. It was great experience, and there was no risk of her screwing up and costing us the game because we were so far ahead. Not that she would screw up; she was great. But a father worries.

Anyway, the varsity games were normally before the JV games. As Ella's game was wrapping up, I'd see our friends Dan and Amy, whose daughter was on JV. As I mentioned, Dan and Amy were using the same pool company we were, but they had started the process much earlier. They had permits, the land was leveled, the hole was dug, neighbors were yelled at, and the pool had been dropped in. That was weeks ago. But then the work stopped.

Dan gave me updates at every game, but they were never positive. He either didn't hear from John at all, or if he did, John would say they were slammed, but he'd be there any day now. John promised

Dan that once they showed up, they'd bang out the work, and the pool would be ready to use by the end of May.

I went back to my earlier calculations, during which I had deduced it was almost mid-May. It wasn't looking too good for Dan and Amy and certainly did not bode well for us.

***

Wednesday was supposed to be a big surprise for Ella: Alix was coming home from Tulane for the summer, but we hadn't told Ella exactly when. Although she knew Alix was coming home eventually, Ella would have a nice happy surprise when Alix showed up. My memory is shot, and I always screw up surprises, so I kept asking Cali when Alix was coming home.

She would look around urgently for a sign of Ella and whisper to me loudly, "Lower your voice! Remember, it's a surprise. She's coming home on Wednesday, May 12. *Don't* screw it up."

Then two nights ago, at dinner, Ella had told Cali she needed more summer clothing.

Cali asked, "What are you worried about? When Alix comes home on Wednesday night, you'll have all the clothes you need."

That whole sentence seemed to take ten minutes. In that time, I could see where the train was headed and was waving and bugging my eyes out at Cali, who took no notice.

"Great, thanks a lot," Ella said, disappointed about the ruined surprise.

Cali thought she'd been talking about the clothes and couldn't understand what she'd done wrong. Ella loved borrowing Alix's clothing. I explained to Cali that she ruined the surprise. It still wasn't clicking.

A few minutes later, she got it. I think they were cooking her brains a little in those chemo sessions.

Anyway, Alix came home as planned. My in-laws picked her up at JFK since Cali felt lousy and I was at Ella's lacrosse game. After the two-hour drive home from the airport, Cali's parents had logged some quality time with Alix. Now it was my turn to hear about school, New Orleans, her boyfriend, her friends, and everything else. Nonetheless, Cali, without consultation, invited her folks to stay for dinner. To their credit, they declined.

That night, we sat on the couch and Alix streamed the photos from her smartphone to the smart TV. All our appliances were becoming smart. We even had a smart robotic vacuum that had recently been looking at me strangely. Alix scrolled through photos and videos on the big screen, telling us all about her semester, her friends, and her adventures. It was so nice and brought a smile to Cali's face.

CHAPTER 32
Wide Awake and Steaming Mad

On Monday, May 17, 2021, I noted that it was technically more than halfway through the month. I had exercised great patience but felt it was now within reason to reach out to Ed the Engineer. I texted him, asking if he felt we should be expecting the permit this week.

No response.

The next day, I gave Ed a little time to get his day going, then added some courtesy cushion time to let him get around to responding to his previous day's texts. He was an old-timer, after all, and maybe that was his normal procedure. At 2 p.m., I could wait no longer and wanted to text him a few question marks or a dramatic *helloooo??* This would have passively yet aggressively indicated my annoyance but also could have possibly put a strain on our lovely relationship. Instead, I came up with a bullshit follow-up question, asking if I should be checking in with him or the town of Somers, just to keep the dialogue going.

An hour later, he wrote back.

The permit application was just mailed. They should get it shortly.

Cryptic.

I thought he'd already mailed the application and I should be expecting the permit mid-May. Also, "just mailed"? Did that mean two weeks ago or five minutes ago? Not wanting to start evil just yet,

I texted back a "thank you" and asked if it usually took a while after they received it.

He didn't answer.

The *next* day, I didn't give Ed quite the same cushion. Around noon, I texted him, asking if I needed to do anything or just wait to hear from the town.

He didn't reply.

Now I was irritated. I was also wondering if my pool guys had told Ed to drag his ass a bit since they were so backed up and didn't want me to be hounding them yet.

On Thursday, my phone buzzed. I was so excited to see it was Ed calling, I almost dropped the phone in my fish tank. I was cleaning it at the time. My fish tank, not the phone—just to be clear.

Ed said he was mailing me something today. I needed to sign wherever he indicated, write a check to the town for $200, and drop everything off at the building department office in Somers. Ed seemed like he was eager to get off the phone, so I said "thanks," and we hung up.

I immediately thought of a million things I wanted to ask him, like, "What are you mailing me today and is it the same or different than what you said you already mailed Tuesday?" And "I thought you took care of everything permit-related, and I didn't have to drop anything off in person, which is part of the reason I paid you so much?" Also, "How much longer will it take after this, what did you accidentally leave out that will require more paperwork, and what are your greatest hopes and fears, Ed?"

The day's other noteworthy occurrence was technically the next day at 2 a.m. That was when I burst into Hunter's bedroom and lost my shit on him, vomiting up everything I had been trying to keep at bay since before he even got home from college.

I was in bed that night, wide awake and steaming mad. I was so frustrated. Hunter had always been such an amazing kid. We'd been best buds, but I believed it was in a healthy way. I had no delusions. I was still his dad. But until recently, we'd often gotten along like brothers. We were just on the same wavelength and absorbed so much of each other's personalities, we would often say the same random thing at the same time and then look at each other in surprise and crack up.

Hunter is smart, funny, handsome, charismatic, and nice. I love introducing any of my three kids to people because I'm so proud, and they handle themselves so well. Once, at my niece's bat mitzvah, Cali's brother Sean introduced Hunter to his friend John R. I already knew John, who is very successful, very funny, and has a great bullshit detector. Hunter, who was seventeen at the time, looked John in the eye and shook his hand, saying it was nice to meet him.

I stepped away to grab a drink. When I came back, Hunter and John were still talking and laughing. I listened in as they spoke about girls, Ohio State, and football. Then John began to give Hunter some advice about school, explaining how important good grades were to a prospective employer. John said he always scanned an applicant's résumé for their GPA first before he read the rest of it. I hung back, not wanting to interfere and glad for the advice Hunter was getting.

John grabbed me later. "Hey, man. Your son is awesome. Do you know how many kids his age are just gigantic pieces of shit? They can't manage to make eye contact or give a proper handshake, much less carry on a conversation the way Hunter just did. What a kid. Great job."

I was flattered, but I already knew this. Hunter was special. Even though there was a sadly low bar out there, apparently, based on John's experience.

Well, John wasn't just blowing smoke up my ass because any time I ran into him again through Sean or on occasion via a group text, he would ask about Hunter.

That's the kind of kid Hunter is ... *was?*

Either way, it was breaking my heart to see Hunter in this funk. I was equally mad, sad, and confused. Parenting him was always so easy, and it was like a different kid had come home from college and was inhabiting my beloved son's room. And again, I still didn't know which angle to take: strictness and rules, or compassion and passivity.

That night, I was leaning toward strictness and rules. I was awake and angry at 2 a.m. I was spending all this mental and physical energy on Hunter when I had so many other things on my plate.

Fuck it, I thought. *I'm not hanging on to this. He's definitely awake right now. I'm going in there.*

I got up, stormed down the hallway, gave a perfunctory knock on his closed door, and let myself in. Always a risky move with a teenage son. Hunter was lying propped up on his bed, laptop open, and headphones on. He looked up, surprised to see me at this hour. And in my underwear. Whoops.

He slid one side of his headphones off and paused whatever he was watching. "What's up, *Padre*?"

I told him what was up. That I was lying awake all night, worried about him. That I didn't know what the fuck was going on with him, and I was terrified that my beloved boy was possibly taking a permanent turn for the worse. I told him how angry it made me every day, as each hour ticked by and he was still asleep. How torn I was between feeling bad for him and being pissed that he didn't have a job or internship. How badly I felt that COVID had stolen his junior year, and his mom was sick, but how mad I was that he wasn't rising above it all.

I was all over the place. I wasn't even sure what I was saying, but I had to get it all out. I was yelling, crying, pacing his room. He must have thought I was a maniac. Poor bastard was just trying to watch some YouTube videos in the privacy of his own room.

I finally finished my rant and stood there, panting.

He just looked at me, then said, "I don't know what to tell you. I'm not good. I don't know what to do, but I don't feel any passion for life right now, and I am scared to death of finishing my senior year and having to go out into the real world."

Ugh.

I softened immediately. I gave him a hug, which he welcomed. I held him for a while, my big little boy. We agreed to talk more at a reasonable hour.

I went back to my room and fell asleep with ease.

★★★

Our late-night conversation aside, I still spent Friday morning silently simmering in anger as I worked and Hunter slept the day away. He came down to eat at some point that afternoon. I was in my office, but I heard Cali begin to interrogate him about his plans for the summer. He was hemming and hawing, and I finally couldn't hold out any longer. I went into the kitchen under some false pretense. I picked up a glass and inspected it carefully as Hunter began to get more defensive with Cali.

I inserted myself into the discussion. "Hunter, you can't keep operating like you did in high school. You can't just lean on good looks and charisma. You've got to work at life."

Hunter has always been very smart and, as a result, never had to work very hard. In high school, he crushed his classes through natural smarts and made up for any shortcomings by turning on the charm with his teachers. He would do month-long assignments the night before they were due. He aced his test about *The Great Gatsby* without ever reading a page. He crushed his ACT and SAT without any prep or special tutoring. It all just came naturally, but in my judgment, he was operating at 80 percent.

I always thought, *If this kid turns it up a notch, there will be no stopping him.*

I had assumed his *modus operandi* continued into college, so for the past three years, I imagined that he wasn't working incredibly hard and was continuing to game the system. I told him that now.

Hunter replied, "I know you think that about me, but that isn't true anymore. Sure, when I first got to school, I'd try to talk my way through a freshman class or two. But I quickly learned that wasn't going to fly. I work hard at school, Dad, and my grades show it."

His GPA was a 3.6, so I couldn't argue with that.

It suddenly occurred to me that I was wrong—mostly. Perhaps there was still some truth to my perception of him, but it wasn't fair to assume Hunter was half-assing it *all* the time. I apologized for my inaccurate judgment of him and said I was glad we'd cleared it up. Still, I was tired of pussyfooting around with him. There was no way I'd make it through this summer with him sleeping all day and otherwise lazing about.

"Hunter, let's make this simple. What do you need from us, as your parents? Should we keep pushing you to get up at a normal hour, take better care of yourself, and to look for an internship or job? Or are we supposed to just leave you alone to do whatever you want?"

Hunter had already said he was a grown-ass adult four times in his earlier conversation with Cali, which, to me, was a sure sign of someone who was not completely confident about their adulthood. You don't hear me shouting at age forty-eight that I'm an adult. Well, not often.

He wouldn't, or couldn't, answer my most direct questions and began to get choked up. Then he began to cry. "You guys don't know what I went through this year!" he sobbed.

That was true. I didn't. I assumed COVID had put a damper on the festivities, but otherwise, I imagined him sleeping late, cramming in some schoolwork, and pausing his partying and video games only to welcome a healthy rotation of young coeds into his lair.

Hunter explained that although there had indeed been many good times, he was also often incredibly depressed. He'd be alone in his room for long periods of time, occasionally felt he didn't fit in completely with any one group, was down about the state of the world in general, and then got whacked in the head with the bonus news that his mom was sick.

I could identify with all that. I had been feeling the same way. But I hadn't realized it was so bad for Hunter.

He was weeping now, sitting at the kitchen table, having spilled everything. We let him cry and just stood there, looking at him, looking at each other. He eventually grew quiet. He was an empty vessel now, his head down, and his long hair hanging down his face and pooling on the table.

Cali was sitting at the table, crying. I was standing with my back up against the counter, still holding the glass I had been pretending to inspect. I put it down, carefully. The room was so quiet, it was deafening. I wondered where the cats were.

In the past, Hunter had mentioned on occasion that he would be interested in therapy. But whenever I offered to find someone, he would be on the upswing of his mood curve and politely decline the offer. He'd brought it up several times since he'd been home though, and I asked now if he wanted to give it a try. We had already done some research and found someone, and she could see him the following Tuesday. Hunter was into it.

We made an agreement. We would stay off his ass at least until his appointment on Tuesday. Of course, not everything would be resolved in his first session, but we would take baby steps and start with that.

It was a load off all our minds. Hunter knew we would leave him alone for the next few days, and we knew we could stop stewing over things for now. It was a temporary cease-fire.

I also felt good having cleared up my misconceptions about his work ethic and getting everything out on the table about how he'd been feeling.

That evening, Hunter joined me and Cali for Ella's lacrosse game at John Jay Cross River High School. It had been a warm day and was still beautiful in the afternoon. The game was at 6 p.m., so we took the soft-top off the Jeep and headed over early. There was a pizza place right by the high school. We sat outside and ate some slices and made light conversation. It was the first time since Hunter had gotten home that there wasn't an underlying tension between all of us.

Although the Somers team was excellent, John Jay was rumored to be better. It was an exciting game, and it was close the whole time. Somers squeezed out a win in the end, and Ella didn't get to play.

By the time we got back in the Jeep, the air was colder. The soft-top roof was too much of a pain in the ass to put back up, so we drove home with the cold air whipping our faces while the heat, which we cranked up, blasted our legs.

Back home, it was dark. Cali went inside, so Hunter and I worked to put the top back up on the Jeep. We worked mostly in silence, occasionally giving each other simple directions. We had done this before.

We worked well together.

CHAPTER 33
Friends and Family

On Tuesday, May 26, we received the paperwork from Ed the Engineer. I excitedly opened the manila envelope, carefully unfolded the large engineering drawing inside, and immediately laughed, shaking my head. I was sure everything was up to all the latest technical requirements, but, essentially, the guy had drawn a pool right onto our existing survey and put an official-looking stamp on it.

Cali wrote a check to the town and brought the drawing and our signed documents in herself. I could have, but the town building supervisor was the father of a girl from Alix's former soccer team, and we wanted him to see Cali.

Don't make me say it.

Okay, fine, we were hoping they'd get to talking, and naturally he would also notice her physical appearance. Cali would work into the conversation that she was sick, and we were trying to get the pool done this summer because, hey, you only live once. Maybe he'd feel badly and push it through. This was all unspoken, but we definitely both had the same thought.

I never said we were good people.

That evening, Ella's lacrosse game was away at Yorktown. The school has a strange layout and it is a long walk from the car to the stands of the Yorktown field. Cali's legs were hurting on the walk, and I could tell she was in pain during the entire game, even though she wouldn't admit it.

We had friends in Yorktown. Their daughter played lacrosse, so we figured we'd see them. Simon and Livia.

In the summer of 2017, while the kids were away at camp, I'd gotten antsy and booked a last-minute trip for Cali and me. Nothing fancy; we were going to the Sagamore up on Lake George for the Fourth of July weekend. I figured we'd laze about the pool and lake and have a nice private getaway.

The night I booked the trip, Cali mentioned it to Brenda who then told Cali her good friends Simon and Livia were going to be there at the same time. She would let them know and give them our number. We were sure to hit it off.

I immediately investigated the Sagamore's cancellation policy, but it was too late to make any changes without penalty. We were locked in. I spent the next two weeks dreading our upcoming trip. Although we knew Simon and Livia from other gatherings enough to recognize them, we didn't *know* them. They were friends of friends, which was the case for pretty much anyone we knew. I wasn't looking for new friends. I wasn't even looking for my old ones. My plan, when we saw them, was to politely drop into the early conversation that we were very excited to have some alone time and hope they got the hint. Still, I wasn't excited about awkwardly bumping into them around the resort afterward.

Cali and I arrived at the Sagamore after a three-hour drive. We checked in and immediately changed for the pool. Before we went down, I told Cali to text Livia right away so we could meet them and get it over with. I had already spent too much energy dreading this situation. Cali's phone dinged back immediately, telling us they were poolside. Livia provided the coordinates.

The place was more crowded than I'd hoped, and there were way more kids than I'd expected. There were kids bouncing off everything. Not sure what I was thinking, booking this as a romantic getaway. It was a family resort on the Fourth of July; of course it would be crowded and crawling with kids. Not everyone went to sleepaway camp. We got to the pool and managed to find two seats that had just opened. It was midafternoon, and some people were calling it quits after a day in the sun. We put our things down, and I suggested we go find these two right away so we could try to enjoy ourselves. We'd say hello, compare mutual acquaintances, make mild small talk, and fuck off.

It was a multileveled pool deck, so we worked our way over to where Livia said they were lounging. We approached and recognized it was, indeed, the Simon and Livia we knew from here and there. There was one small problem. They were both out cold. We stood at the foot of their lounge chairs, looking down at them.

Cali said, "We'll come back later."

I said, "I am not checking their nap status every half hour while I wallow in misery. We're doing this now." Then I kicked one of the lounge chairs.

Livia jumped awake to find the sun eclipsed by a giant, hairy stranger. Her face did not mask her confusion. Then she saw past me and recognized Cali. She elbowed Simon awake. They both sat up.

We talked a bit and agreed to meet later at the bar. Screw it, they seemed okay.

We wound up spending three hours with them. Simon was British, funny, and fascinating. He was in advertising and had tons of funny stories. And Livia and Cali were kindred spirits.

We spent the next few days with them. We even rented a boat together for the day, and I caught the biggest trout of my life. We ate it at the restaurant together that night and fed half the waitstaff with the leftovers. We sat on the main lawn and watched the fireworks afterward. A few dozen boats dotted the darkened lake with their lights as we watched the show.

They have become good friends of ours—another perfect example of me being completely wrong about a situation. You'd think I'd have learned by now.

So, when we saw them at Ella's game, I pulled Simon aside. I explained Hunter had been down about his mom and rudderless when it came to facing the real world and a career. In lieu of an internship, I was reaching out to some of my friends in various fields to see if they could spend some time with him. Anything from an hour lunch to a week in the office to, ideally, a full internship, if so inclined.

Simon put his hand up and stopped me. He said, "Anything you need, mate. Have him reach out to me."

People. Underrated?

★ ★ ★

On Saturday, May 29, Cali's parents came over. My niece Emma brought her girlfriend for us to meet for the first time. Cali warned me to be on my best behavior because it was a big deal for Emma. It was pouring out, but I still insisted on grilling. Mostly so I could be alone outside. I put on a raincoat and stood there, the steam rising as the cold raindrops pelted the hot grill cover. I could hear the conversation and laughs in the kitchen through the window. Cali seemed happy. I smiled to myself as I tried to get the steaks to cook properly in these unusual conditions.

Later, after dinner, we sat around talking in the kitchen. Cali took off her bandana to show everyone her current hair situation. At this point, she looked like a baby ostrich. Mostly bald and gray with a few pitiful wisps here and there. Cali's mom began crying.

As soon as the bandana came off, Big Al immediately walked out of the kitchen and into the dining room. I waited a minute and then followed him in. It was still a little light out, and the rain had let up. He was staring out the front window at nothing. I stood a few feet away by the side window and spoke to his back. "I cut back those thick thorn bushes that were coming through the fence."

He turned his head to look at the fence through the side window.

I kept looking out the window. "Yeah, they were really growing, so I cut back a four-foot swath on the other side of the fence. Almost passed out halfway through though."

He looked back out the front window and said, "Good job. You gotta be careful though. Don't push it."

I agreed I wouldn't push it. I told him I saw a big deer with velvet antlers out front the other day. He told me about a bobcat that had been coming by his place.

Eventually, we went back into the kitchen and joined the others. Cali had put her bandana back on.

★ ★ ★

Hunter had lunch with Simon on Sunday. Simon once ran a large advertising firm and was later CEO of a cannabis company. He had a lot of interesting stories and advice on what to do when life kicks you in the balls. When Hunter returned, he seemed different than he had been lately. He was energized, even had a little sparkle in his eye. Hunter liked Simon.

Simon later texted me that the feeling was mutual. *I'm gonna make that little wanker my pet project*, he wrote.

That night, I went out to dinner with Alix and Ella. It was strange sitting inside at a crowded restaurant. As nice as it was to see some return to normalcy, I also felt all the old irritations coming back. My mind raced as the walls closed in a bit.

Who lets their kid run around like that? Hasn't it been a while since we ordered? Is that guy wearing flip-flops in a restaurant? Does this lady really need to walk so close to our table?

I missed my cocoon. It was much easier ordering contactless delivery, saying "thank you" through the video doorbell, and eating at a snack table while streaming *Parks and Recreation*.

We got home to find Cali and Hunter in the kitchen. Cali's hair was wispy, but until now all those wisps had looked even when they were pulled back and sticking out the back of a baseball cap. Now, even the wisps looked spotty poking out of a hat or bandana.

She handed me a pair of scissors and said, "Just cut it."

As the kids stared, I carefully snipped off the length in the back, so any hair now stopped just at her neckline. It still looked wild with no covering but would look less uneven with a hat. Cali bunched up the hair I'd cut off and made a fake mustache with it. She was yukking it up for us. Even though we were laughing, it was a somber moment.

CHAPTER 34
June

I drove Cali to the beginning of her fifth round of chemo on Tuesday, June 1. The schedule was shifted out a day from Monday because of Memorial Day weekend. She was now officially past the two-thirds point and it felt like we were making progress. Ella had an eye doctor appointment nearby, so she came with us. I dropped Cali off and took Ella to her appointment, where she got her final fitting for contact lenses. We got back home by 10 a.m., where I jumped into work after the long weekend.

At 11:30 a.m., Mitchell called. He was walking down the city street and huffing while he spoke. He was irate. "Why the fuck are so many people still wearing masks?" he asked.

Was he asking *me*? I didn't know the answer. I suspected some people weren't vaccinated yet, so they were wearing masks. I also figured some were vaccinated, but since there were so many who weren't getting vaccinated and not wearing masks, they felt it was better to be safe than sorry. Maybe some were vaccinated but still felt a sense of security a mask provided by protecting them from the outside world. It occurred to me I hadn't even gotten a cold for the last year, and I might keep the mask going in certain situations, like on a crowded subway or my living room couch. Plus, there were new variants erupting in various parts of the world, so who knew what was happening?

In addition to the mask thing, Mitchell was bent out of shape about gas prices and inflation and how hard it was to find people to work in the factory. He had a lot of concerns and rightfully so. Business was off a bit, and the sooner the world got back to normal, the sooner people would start wearing makeup and lipstick and going out to stores and buying product, which in turn would cause our numbers to pick back up. We were, after all, manufacturers of cosmetic packaging.

Still, it felt like Mitchell had just mainlined triple-espressos with Tucker Carlson. On top of his manic mood, his phone was breaking up. Mitchell finished his frantic report of everything wrong in the world, and there was an awkward moment of silence. I didn't have much to offer in the way of opinion, and I certainly didn't have control over any of the things he was saying. Yet, I still felt guilty somehow for enjoying the new way of the world.

But I had other things to worry about, some of which *were* under my control. Work deadlines, projects, Zoom meetings, phone calls, emails, reports, customer relationships, competitors, an internal team to manage, and a million other work-related things. I had a sick wife, my own shaky health, a thick schedule of doctor appointments for us both, a mortgage, college payments, this pool nonsense, and millions of things to do around the house. I had a nonexistent college search and driving lessons for Ella, my relationship with Alix and concern about her general well-being, a sad and listless son who was currently lost at sea, one cat that was on prescription food for a small pee hole, and another cat that liked to poop on his own tail. You don't want more detail on the cat thing.

It was hard to get back to work after that call. It just all seemed so futile. Even if I overcame everything within my power, it wasn't going to be enough. It was never going to be enough. I felt overwhelmed.

Just then, my dad called my cell. I picked up, wondering if something was wrong in Florida since it was the middle of a workday and an unusual time to call. I imagined some terrible news about my mother, or maybe the condo clubhouse was closed for renovations.

Luckily, he was just saying hello and checking on Cali. I appreciated the call but had zero motivation to make idle chitchat and even less ability to fake it. He must have sensed it because he asked if I was okay. I was not. As I began to explain, I started crying a little. I felt embarrassed at first. There's a natural tendency to act like I have my shit together when speaking with my dad. But it was good to let go. It felt honest, and my dad appreciated it. He listened and didn't go overboard with the advice. I felt better afterward.

While I was speaking with my father, Hunter left for therapy. He waved goodbye as he passed my office and headed into the garage.

Well, we were all just having a great time, weren't we?

At 1 p.m., I left to pick Cali up from treatment.

That day was also my grandmother's birthday. I thought about "Nana Ruth" as I drove. Ruth is gone now, as are all my amazing grandparents, but I like to keep track of their birthdays and anniversaries and other milestones so I can give them a mental shout out and spend a moment remembering them on those occasions.

I have zero recollection of the facts, timing, and accuracy of what I'm about to tell you, and I don't care to look it up or research it, so here's my loose version.

Nana Ruth and Popi Rip were my father's parents. At some point, Ruth had breast cancer. She went through treatment and had a double mastectomy. I was young, too young at the time to understand what was happening, and I'm sure I wasn't given a lot of information either. Rightfully so. I vaguely remember finding her fake boob inserts on her night table once and squeezing them without comprehension, so I was that young. Many years later, it dawned on me what they were, and I had the sudden urge to wash my hands. And brain.

Years later, Ruth developed cancer in her throat and palette. She went through treatment. They performed surgery and removed her palette and other internal facial parts, which essentially caved in the left half of her face and throat. This was around 1984 or 1985. I remember because I recall the concern leading up to my bar mitzvah that she wasn't going to live to be there for it.

I'm sure I am getting a lot of this wrong, but it's irrelevant. The point is, Ruth survived and made it to my big, fat, awkward bar mitzvah. She wore large tinted sunglasses and a huge, floppy white hat to cover her features and danced and celebrated like there was no tomorrow. Which she knew there might not be, having stood so close to the precipice.

Ruth developed other maladies as time went on. Through it all, she was a tough, loving, powerhouse of a woman. I took note of this as an impressionable young lad. Equally interesting was how her husband—my hard-assed, broken-nosed, cigar-smoking, old-school, football coach Popi Rip—handled it. Imagine if Vince Lombardi had a love child with Bill Clinton. That was The Ripper. Tough as nails but lovable and charismatic. He softened with each hurdle and grew ever more loving and caring for his Ruthie. It was a powerful example to witness.

I've always dabbled in art, and for their fiftieth anniversary, I drew a portrait of Ruth and Rip. I presented it to them, expecting high praise and appreciation. Ruth took one look and made her signature noise of disapproval ("uchhh") as she closed her eyes, shrugged, and turned her head away like a kid in front of a plate of liver. I was momentarily crushed. I was proud of that drawing and it was almost an exact likeness. But Ruth never minced words, and she seemed displeased.

She went on to explain she appreciated the gesture, but she just hated her appearance. I took a good look at her. Ruth's skin was permanently tanned. It was leathery and wrinkled from many long-ago cigarettes and years of the harsh Florida sun. Her white hair was cropped short. She had tens of bracelets running up both thin arms because she refused to *not* display gifts from her grandchildren, and for some reason we kept buying her bracelets. The left side of her face and throat were all concave. Her cheek was sunken, and the eye there drooped and watered. Her voice was nasal, and she couldn't pronounce certain consonants. But I swear I didn't see any of that. It was just Nana Ruth. She was beautiful to me, and I loved her with all my heart. I explained that to her.

She shrugged and again said, "Uchhh."

Rip took her hand and said softly, "Ah, Ruthie, you look great. We'll hang the drawing over there." He winked at me.

I think back on that now and realize I learned a lot from those two. Cali's toughness and attitude are so much like Ruth's. Cali, ever concerned about cancer's impact on her appearance, her weight, and, most importantly to her, her hair. Me, like Rip, just being glad my wife is alive, thinking she is beautiful no matter what, and trying to reassure her.

I wish Ruth and Rip never had to go through all that, but I am glad I had those positive lessons as a kid.

★ ★ ★

My buddy Jacko invited me to Game 5 of the Knicks playoffs. He and my brother Bryan had bonded over the Knicks during our last ice-fishing trip. He had three tickets and certainly wanted Bryan there, so he invited the two of us. New Gregg said "yes" before Old Gregg could get involved. Plus, I wanted to hang with my brother. And Jacko. Although I was hesitant to leave Cali for the night.

So, on Wednesday, I drove for twenty minutes to the local train station. I parked and walked to the train. The train was late arriving, but it was midafternoon, so it wasn't too crowded. The train ride was eighty-eight minutes. It got more and more crowded as we neared the city. No one sat next to me, although I cringed in anticipation at each stop.

We arrived, and I shuffled along behind all the other disembarking passengers into Grand Central. I exited onto street level and stepped into a city I hadn't seen in over a year.

Strangely, my last time in the city had also been spent at Madison Square Garden. Things had just started cooking with COVID on March 10, 2020, but it was still something that was happening to other people in other places. Like SARS or bird flu or Ebola and all the other past threats, it didn't seem real. Whatever we were hearing in the news in 2020, though, concerned me enough to consider skipping the Allman Brothers concert that night. I didn't skip it, but everything took a turn that day. The city shut down soon thereafter, and I hadn't been back since.

Before then, I'd commuted regularly into the city. I loved and hated the place. Some nights, I'd come out of a bar and see the Christmas lights and love the feel of the city buzzing around me. Other days, I'd be sweating in the sweltering summer heat, swimming through the stench of hot garbage, and would have to fight the urge to punch a slow-moving tourist in the neck.

Either way, it was nice to be back. And coming to this Knicks game was something I'd never have agreed to if I had to be back in the city the very next morning for work.

Things seemed different though. There had been a rash of homelessness recently, and crime was rising. There were random stabbings on the subway and muggings in broad daylight. There was a reported rise in anti-Semitism. There were violent protests. I found myself looking over my shoulder more often than usual on the walk to meet Bryan and Jacko. Many storefronts were closed, and was it my imagination, or did the city seem dirtier?

After we chowed down at Wolfgang's, and I had imbibed one or four Manhattans, we walked to the Garden. It was absolutely packed. We waited in a huge line to get into the building. A massive surge of people was chaotically breaking off into lines as we approached the turnstiles. Then we walked a bit and waited on another ridiculously long line inside to enter our gate. Again, just a huge crowd with no organization. There were people cutting in front of, bumping into, and jostling us. It was wall-to-wall people in orange and blue, shouting, yelling, chanting. The air was heavy with the sweet stink of alcohol and weed. I was overwhelmed as we shuffled closer and closer to the entrance. We finally made it through and took the escalators up and up and up until we reached our section. I shoehorned myself into the tiny seat, my legs uncomfortably pressed against my brother on the left, a large man to my right, and the seats in front of me.

The place was rocking. The Knicks had to win tonight to stay alive against the Hawks as they were down 3–1 before this return home. People were happy to be out. They were drunk, high, cursing, and yelling. It was loud. The crowd stood up for every shot or big play, so we had to decide to either miss seeing the play or stand up and sit down repeatedly. If we stood up, people behind us would yell at us, though, so for me, it was a night of doing drunken squats and making big decisions.

The Knicks fell apart, which also put a damper on the evening. Even my brother, who is a huge Knicks fan and general sports enthusiast, turned to me at the end of the game and said, "I would've rather been on my couch."

I felt the same way, and this was only exacerbated by my subway trek back to Grand Central, where I encountered a glowing green puddle of vomit, and an eighty-eight-minute train ride home.

I was equally glad to have gotten out, though, and to spend some time with Jacko and Bryan. It was a toss-up.

★ ★ ★

June continued. Time was moving aggressively, as if Earth had started spinning faster because it felt close to the end of this COVID situation and wanted out.

Things were cooking out there in the world. Vaccination was more common than not. Infection rates were dropping. Restaurants were opening and regulations were being lifted. Live music and other performances were being announced. People were frantically booking vacations and making plans. A sinister new COVID variant was poking its evil head out in Europe and elsewhere, but it hopefully wouldn't become a factor here. India was having a rough go of it lately, I heard.

Each day ripped by like wildfire for me. Wake up, grab a coffee in the kitchen, hit my home office, work through the morning. Eat lunch at my desk, work through the afternoon, do nothing for an hour before dinner. Eat dinner, watch something on the tube with Cali, go upstairs. Lie in bed, watch something else, go to sleep. Repeat. The only change was when I had to drive Cali somewhere.

Ella was going to high school parties seemingly every night. Her grade partied harder than Hunter's and Alix's combined. Her lacrosse season had concluded in a heartbreaking loss in the championship game. It was an exciting season though, and I was proud of her. She had handled coming off the bench with class. She repeatedly stepped out of her comfort zone socially, and she was killing it in school.

On the flip side, she still had a lot of high school friend bullshit drama, she was absolutely terrified of her impending road test at the end of the month, and her OCD was so bad, it was almost paralyzing at times.

Alix seemed great. She was even-keeled and happy. Things were cool with her boyfriend from Tulane, who was back home in Chicago. They seemed to have things well in hand. Alix worked out like a maniac, saw her friends on occasion, and was interning for Cali's sister at Designs That Donate. She was incredibly independent, sometimes annoyingly so, but at the same time, I was proud of her.

Alix's boyfriend flew in and spent a long weekend with us. Blake's a nice Jewish kid from a nice Chicago suburb. Pre-med. Parents own a deli. You can't make up a better biography. He had a nice visit here. They did their own thing and hung out with us just enough. They hiked, Blake met Alix's friends from home, and they explored the Hudson Valley region. One night, we took him to my favorite BBQ and beer joint. We sat outside and had a nice time. I might have gotten him drunk.

Peer pressure, kids. Don't give in.

Hunter was up and down. He'd lost touch with many of his high school friends and only got together with one or two. But he was incredibly tight with his one buddy, Cameron, and they spent a lot of quality time together. Hunter was still sleeping late each day but seemed to really be valuing his therapist's advice. She suggested he set a goal to be asleep by midnight and awake by 9 a.m., and he listened. He'd been setting his alarm for nine, but then hit snooze because he said he didn't know what to do once he got out of bed. That was tough to hear, and I vowed to make a few more calls on his behalf to find him some purpose and get his spark back. It was breaking my heart to see him like this.

My parents had been incredibly supportive and continued to be. My dad texted me practically every day to see how Cali was doing.

And how I was doing. My mom was great too. I could tell they felt for us and were genuinely concerned. I imagine they felt a bit powerless as well, being so far away and unable to help. Not that we would have let them help if they were here, anyway, but I got it. They sent flowers, called the house, and checked in with regularity.

Cali's parents were hanging in there. Cali still spoke to her mom several times a day, in between speaking to her mom several times a day. And at least twice a week, her parents would stop by and commiserate in the kitchen with Cali. I'd pop out of my office to say hello. Cali kept her mask on when someone visited because she still couldn't be vaccinated, but we finally convinced her parents to remove theirs.

Big Al would swing by toward the end of each week and text me to come out and meet him in the driveway, where he'd hand me a large bag of bagels. We would make some small talk and hug it out, and then he would head off. We didn't really need someone to bring us bagels, but it was something he wanted to do, and it was nice.

★ ★ ★

On a boiling hot Sunday, Cali came down and tore her bandana off in frustration. What was left of her hair was a patchy mess. "Buzz it," she ordered.

I got my clippers, and we went out on the deck. The heat slapped us like a giant, wet hand as Cali settled into a chair. Sorry for the gross word, but we were instantly *moist*. My shirt was already sticking to my man-boobs. I asked Cali one last time if she was sure about this. She once again gave her consent. I buzzed away. It didn't take very long, but we both got quiet as I pulled each errant strand away, buzzed it off, and wiggled my fingers to unstick them from my sweaty hand.

When I was done, I adjusted the clipper settings and gave her a nice once-over. Then I cleaned up around her ears and the back of her neck. Cali ran her hand over her fuzzy, sweaty head. She smiled, maybe feeling free of those last wisps. What was left was a salt-and-pepper fuzzy buzz cut. Mostly salt.

I thought she looked incredible.

CHAPTER 35
Perspective

It was August 2009, and the evening began at Frankie Rowland's with pineapple martinis at the bar. Frankie's is still one of my favorite steakhouses, and it is not in New York City or Chicago. It is in downtown Roanoke, Virginia, next to a Subway sandwich shop.

Our factory is a short drive from downtown Roanoke. I use the term *downtown* loosely. It is a slowly expanding five square blocks of restaurants, bars, art galleries, bookstores, coffee shops, and, on Wednesdays, an outdoor produce market. The city is something Jack Reacher may happen upon in his travels, and somewhere he may find trouble too. Walking one block in the wrong direction puts you literally and figuratively on the wrong side of the tracks. The city has been struggling for years to emerge from its cocoon as something else, something better. It gets close and then falls back, repeating the cycle but making progress each time.

Mitchell has contributed greatly to the Taubman Museum of Art, a hulking modern spaceship perched on the edge of the otherwise brick-and-mortar anchor. There are colleges and universities nearby. There are factories nearby. There is a medical facility nearby. There are also miles of open country nearby. And there is poverty to be found in the corners. Each of these groups competes for access to the small downtown area. Sometimes they take turns. Sometimes they overlap.

The result is completely unpredictable. There are nights when you can literally hear crickets chirping downtown. Some nights, it feels like a wild college party has spread throughout the streets and bars. Other nights, it is downright scary. Usually, it is somewhere in between.

When I visit the factory, I stay at the Hotel Roanoke Conference Center. The large Tudor-style hotel was built in 1882 on a wheat field, just overlooking the railroad tracks. As travelers began stopping there on their journeys elsewhere, the hotel and city both grew. The area was so promising that even during the Great Depression, the railroad invested $225,000 in a seventy-five-room wing. That's the equivalent of over $4 million today.

The hotel has a rich history of ownership, renovations, and décor changes, but the most important might have been in 1995, when they reopened after a $5 million renovation that included a glass-enclosed walking bridge from the hotel. The bridge crosses over the railroad tracks below and delivers visitors directly into downtown Roanoke, opening the city to visitors and travelers alike. That was around the same time I started working at Arkay and around the same time we broke ground on our new state-of-the-art factory in Roanoke.

Arkay slowly phased all production out of our expensive Long Island facility and into Roanoke. It was, and still is, a cutting-edge manufacturing facility. In fact, we've been told by auditors it is the cleanest they've ever seen. It was a perfect move for us to remain competitive against China and others. The only downside was we were printers, really, and the convenience of a customer being able to pop out to Long Island for a one-day press approval was the main sacrifice of closing and selling the building in Long Island, aside from losing some good people. But a handful of people were at the right point in their lives and decided to relocate, so that was good.

Before our customers' budgetary travel restrictions, COVID limitations, and my own general desire to travel less, I used to go down there a lot. It was often enjoyable. Initially, we used a small twin-prop Piper Navajo plane that Mitchell's father owned, which is a terrifying story for another day. Eventually, there was a direct flight from LaGuardia to Roanoke, which made it easier to pop down with a customer. Normally, I'd fly down late afternoon, have dinner with the customer, show up as early as possible for the press run the next day, and get out of there on that afternoon's flight. If it wasn't possible to finish in a day, I'd spend two nights.

Either way, it was the perfect amount of time to get to know my customer better, have a nice meal or fun night with them, take care of business at the factory, and get out of Dodge. I didn't know what I'd do with myself if I had three nights down there.

Eric Simon didn't either. The team at Arkay had discovered this tough Long Island kid's impeccable eye for color and savant-like ability to manipulate digital files that would always result in the best printing outcome. When we built the factory down South, he took the opportunity offered to head down there. He eventually took the lead in the printing and prepress departments and later became part of the small-team management approach that Arkay successfully applied. Either way, he was my go-to guy in Virginia when I needed to get something done.

It had been a difficult cultural transition when we initially built that factory. Our brash sense of New *Yawk* urgency and frank communication was lost on the rural Virginian employees. No judgment, but it was like running quickly into the water. You'd sprint down the beach, then when you hit the water, you'd be pumping your legs just as hard, if not harder, but you weren't going as fast and were exerting *more* effort. It took a while to build a culture of urgency and attention to detail we took for granted in New York.

Eric had been part of that growth. After several frustrating press runs before Eric was promoted, I'd had enough. We would show up ungreeted, I would run around the plant looking for someone to give me the status, and we'd wait for hours without any updates for the next adjusted press sheet. There was no water, no snacks, nothing. It was maddening. This was back during a tough period when Walter S., our current COO, and Brian H., our current VP of operations, weren't yet directly overseeing the manufacturing operation. I wrote up a manifesto explaining how things should be handled down there, and so did a few of the other salespeople, including Walter. At the same time, Walter and Brian began running operations, Eric was promoted to supervisor, and the red-carpet treatment was implemented.

After that, I enjoyed my trips to Virginia. I only had to go once every month or two, so it was just the right amount of travel. While there, I always invited some of the guys to join us for dinner with the customer. It was good for them to bond over a fun night before a challenging day on press, during which many designers showed their difficult side and sharp teeth. Building that camaraderie and trust in advance always helped. So normally, I'd have John S., head of quality and all-around good old boy, and Eric, head of the print department, join us.

Most of my customers are women. Back then, there were many package developing engineers who'd come out of Michigan State University, which has one of the only packaging engineering programs in the country. That's my alma mater. And, at the time, those many years ago, we were all young and vibrant. What I'm trying to say is I had a lot of young, fun, female customers from Michigan who loved to party. Eric was helpful in that area as well.

The customer experience was nice. We'd arrive at the small Roanoke airport on a convenient direct flight, hop in a rental car, and drive to the Hotel Roanoke. Upon landing, and during the fifteen-minute drive to the hotel, the customer would see miles of open country, rolling hills, and green mountains. At the right time of year, the pear or cherry trees would be blossoming, highlighting everything with a brilliant white. We would pull up to the Hotel Roanoke and enter another era. The hotel is updated and modernized where it matters but preserved in all the right ways. You can feel the history, minus any shameful parts. Customers would then be checked in by the sweetest and slowest-moving front desk employee with the strongest drawl in the South and handed two homemade chocolate chip cookies. Still warm. I'd usually eat one right away and save the other for a drunken snack later that night.

We would head off to our rooms to get settled and plan to meet downstairs in an hour or so. After a quick nap or shower or time spent frantically answering emails and phone calls, we would meet in the lobby. We would walk out into the sweet, warm Virginia air and casually walk the glass-enclosed bridge crossing over the train tracks and into downtown Roanoke.

There, the customer would be greeted by a small brick city of buildings no more than three stories high, in most cases. Okay, sometimes they were greeted first by a homeless person meandering around the walking bridge exit, but then came the small brick city. The city that wasn't really a city. Not to us New Yorkers. It was cute though. You could see the old and new merge together. There was an antique shop right next to a smoke shop selling psychedelic T-shirts and "smoking devices" on the lower level. There was a chicken-and-waffles joint next to a sleek and modern art gallery. And there, next to a Subway sandwich shop, was the entrance to Frankie Rowland's Steakhouse, surrounded by windows tinted so dark, they were almost opaque.

That was when, after seeing all this charm and beauty, we would enter Frankie's and suddenly be transported to any given steakhouse in New York City, if you ignored the accents and slow service. There was a sleek mahogany bar serving martinis and scotch. Everything was dark wood and black leather. We'd have a drink (or three) and walk to the coveted Table 50 in the back corner. We would sit down to the white tablecloth and fancy cutlery and wait to meet Eric, who was always a few minutes late because he was still working.

Eric was always working. He would arrive and explain they had a unit go down on the press, or they had a hard time matching a color on a run, or someone had called in sick, so he jumped on and ran the press. Whatever the reason, he had been there since 5 a.m. and was now arriving to dinner with a customer at 7 p.m., which, don't forget, was still technically work.

After all the country kitsch and charm anyone could handle, the customer would always light up when Eric showed up. They enjoyed the country vibe, but then felt at home again in the steakhouse and with Eric there.

Eric was a good-looking guy. I'd say "ruggedly handsome" if you put a gun to my head. He had a strong New York accent and a uniquely raspy voice, probably from ripping Marlboro Reds and yelling over the printing presses all day. He smelled faintly of smoke and aftershave and never looked like he truly belonged in his well-tailored suit and button-down shirt. Mostly because of the tattoo of a rose growing out of his open collar and up the side of his neck, which he later had removed. His tattoo was removed, not his neck. I liked it, but I got it. He wanted to look more professional.

This was when the customer was fully sold on Arkay and Roanoke. John was friendly and soft-spoken. Eric spoke plainly and frankly. He was a technical whiz, and his mannerisms lent an air of authenticity to anything he said. He was like the one auto mechanic you could trust, wheeling out from under your car, wiping his oily hands on a rag while explaining what needed to be done. Whatever it was, you'd believe him and you'd do it.

On this particular night, I had Yuko M. with me. She was not one of the young Michigan women I mentioned but rather a young designer who spoke English with a strong Japanese accent. She had a high-profile job at a huge cosmetics company but managed to be very pleasant. She was a cute lady, with her big glasses and blousy shirt dresses, taking pictures of everything and everyone. I wanted her to meet both John and Eric. I hoped we were going to be doing a lot of work for her, and I wanted her to trust the team. Luckily, they were both able to meet us at the bar at Frankie's first, where we each drank one of their famous pineapple martinis. They soaked pineapples in a huge jug of vodka to make a super sweet, crisp, and cold martini. Actually, I would've rather had a regular martini, but it was the specialty.

"Let's have one more before we sit," someone said. Okay, it was me. I said that.

At the table, we felt the martinis kicking in. Yuko took a picture of her silverware, so maybe she was feeling it too. We ordered our steaks and creamed spinach and potatoes au gratin and—

"Can you also bring out the two-pound lobster and just whack it up for us to share?"

I don't know who said that.

We had another drink while we waited for the food. We were drunk. We had fun conversation. Yuko took pictures of me, Eric, John, the ceiling. She was mesmerized, as everyone was, by Eric's story. How he came down here because he couldn't turn down the opportunity. How he worked his ass off but didn't seem to fit in socially. He had a few funny stories about trying to meet people and his dating adventures. "Don't look over there, but I dated that bartender. Oh, and that waitress. She hates me."

We all laughed.

This was my cue to say, "There should be a reality show about you relocating down here."

It was all so charming. I had no idea he was struggling.

The food came, along with a bottle of cabernet. I know next to nothing about wine, except that I like cabernet. Mitchell is my wine expert, so if he isn't down there with me, I choose either a name I recognize or something in the middle of the price list. We crushed two or three bottles easily. We ate steaks. We were full and happy. Yuko was sufficiently entertained and had taken many photos of her steak and our waitress.

We exited Frankie's, squinting in surprise to see it was still light out. It was like coming out of a movie during the day, everything slightly off-kilter for a few moments. We laughed and stumbled two blocks over to 202 Market, a two-story bar that had changed owners and names more times than I can remember.

Reinforcing the unpredictability of the downtown Roanoke scene, the streets and 202 Market were packed. It was a nice Thursday evening, and the crowd seemed friendly and upbeat. One of John's daughters met us there, having already claimed some space at the smoke-filled bar. Virginia didn't ban smoking indoors until December that year, so my clothes would reek of cigarettes after a night out. Also because I'd wind up bumming a few as the night wore on. We ordered drinks. It got darker out. Eventually, the lights dimmed, and country music came on. As if planned—which it was, according to the flyer on the bar that said, "Line dancing at 9"—a group line dance began. We encouraged Yuko and John's daughter to get in there. John's daughter was wearing a black T-shirt and some tight blue jeans. Her hair was pulled back into a ponytail, and she fit right in, which made sense since she lived down there. Yuko was wearing a silky, bright-blue shirtdress and stood out like a sore thumb, all fancy with her glasses and camera. She was having a blast though.

We watched them from the bar and laughed and drank some more. At 10 p.m., the crowd changed a little, but it was still packed. I couldn't put my finger on it, but the vibe was just different. Unbeknownst to us, it was now Karaoke Night. We drank and laughed and drank as we watched people head up on stage and sing mostly country songs. Some were great, and some were terrible, but everyone sang along. Except for me, Eric, and Yuko. We didn't know most of the songs.

Now it was 11 p.m., and we were silly. The perfect storm of steak, sides, vodka, scotch, wine, and now several beers and mixed drinks was brewing in my belly, but I wasn't feeling it yet. I would later. At that point, I was feeling *goood*.

That was when I had the terrible idea to sing "New York State of Mind" to a bar full of drunken hillbillies.

Eric and I took the stage in our Rolex watches and pinstriped suits. We began to sing Billy Joel's song, but aggressively somehow. Singing into each other's faces, laughing, screwing up the lyrics. We were pointing at people and yelling, "I'm in a New York state of mind! *Yeah!*"

No one was amused. No one was singing along.

I pointed at a huge dude with a short-cropped mohawk and a sleeveless flannel shirt, staring at us angrily from the bar. He was flanked by his equally large and menacing buddies. His monstrous arms were folded across his chest. His lips were pursed in an angry straight line.

I yelled, "Sing along, Mohawk!"

He didn't blink. He kept starting at me and slowly shook his head. *No.*

We finished the song to an almost silent bar. There was a smattering of claps from Yuko and one loud "Boo!" from the far back corner. Eric and I stumbled offstage, still laughing but aware of the shift in tone.

We got back to the bar and were met with more angry stares. Mohawk was whispering to one of his buddies and looking over at us.

We got the fuck out of there.

We laughed, stumbling down the street. John and his daughter said goodnight while Eric lit a cigarette. He suggested we go for one more drink. We took Yuko to a hole-in-the-wall bar where Eric hadn't managed to screw any of the waitresses or bartenders yet and ordered three beers.

Eric put his arm around me and said in his gravelly voice, "You're all right, you know that?"

I knew that. The feeling was mutual.

Yuko signed the first press sheet we brought her the next day.

★ ★ ★

Eric died on Thursday, June 16, 2021.

I woke up to separate texts from Mitchell and Brian. After I read them, I let out a sigh of sadness and was relieved when Cali woke up.

She looked at me and asked, "Eric?"

Eric had had a stroke or massive heart attack a few nights prior. He spent the next few days in a medically induced coma on a respirator. His brain had been deprived of oxygen for over ten minutes, which was just too much for him to handle.

Eric, apparently, had run out of things to do in Roanoke years ago. He had faced some dark times a few years back, but I thought he was clean now after getting some help. Maybe he *was* clean … I have no idea.

Some of this wear and tear might have contributed to his shocking and heartbreaking end. I didn't know for sure, and I probably never will. I don't want to, really. It's all too tragic. It was doubly sad because Eric had developed a relationship with a co-worker from Arkay during the last few years and seemed to be finding some happiness and peace. He had recently planted a garden in his yard.

I thought about Eric quite a bit those few days when he'd been in the hospital. The whole team flew down to Roanoke, and I got updates from Mitchell and Brian a few times a day. That morning, after getting what would be the final update, I somberly went downstairs to my office. It was difficult to concentrate, but I fired off a few emails before I found myself scrolling back through the photos on my computer. I found the ones Yuko had sent me way back when. There was me getting off the plane. There was Yuko's steak. Our waitress. Yuko's fork. There was John, smiling with his daughter, and Eric, sweaty in the summer heat of the bar. There was John's daughter and Yuko, line dancing and laughing. And there I was with Eric, up on the stage, the green-and-orange lights reflecting off the smoke-filled room and filling it with an eerie glow. In one, we were singing right into each other's faces. In another one, Eric was pointing at someone, and I was laughing.

Just moments in a life. Flashes of joy just barely grasped by the fingertips in a stress-filled world.

This is what I remember about Eric: He cared about his work. He was the best at what he did. He laughed. He was an *all right guy*.

And he was broken, like so many of us.

I was reminded that everything could change in a heartbeat.

CHAPTER 36
Premature Celebration?

Cali called the town building department about the pool permits. Of course, she knew the woman working there from around town. Her name was Christine, and she had seen Cali driving recently and, gee, she thought something was wrong but didn't want to pry. Cali told her what was going on, and Christine promised Cali she would do everything in her power to push our paperwork through. She emailed us a list of everything missing from our application and made me an appointment with the town building supervisor for Monday, June 21, 2021.

Cancer card played.

So, after dropping Cali at chemo, I drove back up to Somers for my 10 a.m. appointment with the town. I walked through the entrance to the building department, which had been retrofitted with a tiny wooden cubicle surrounded by plexiglass. This allowed visitors inside while preventing evil diseases from permeating the office. It was hot as Hades in there, and I wondered if, ironically, this tiny prison cell was up to code. There was negative air inside the cubicle, and I began sweating immediately as I shuffled through all the paperwork I had accumulated. The building supervisor greeted me with an awkward air of fuzzy recognition—Alix had played soccer with his daughter in high school. Apparently, I hadn't made much of an impression on him, even though I was at every game. But his face lit up when I reminded him I was Cali's husband. We talked a bit about our wives and our daughters and soccer, and, *man*, was I getting dizzy! I was drowning in my own sweat in this torture chamber, but I was trying to be friendly so this guy wouldn't derail our plans.

Of course, I didn't have half the paperwork I needed, so I left with a list of documents to pull together that was longer than what I'd walked in with. And, we apparently had to file a separate application for ConEd to approve the gas line that would extend to the pool heater.

Pool progress delayed. There was no way Cali would be swimming this summer.

The next day, Cali and I pulled into the driveway to see thirty or so of her friends. They were holding signs and cheering, welcoming her home from her last day of chemo.

Technically, Cali would get her final shot the following day. But Brenda had been the one organizing this shindig, and when she realized she couldn't make it Wednesday, I told her to change it to Tuesday. I didn't want this happening without her there, not after all the support she had given Cali.

Cali started crying as we made the turn, and she subsequently took a while to gather herself and get out of the car. She was greeted with hugs and cheers and signs. Someone handed me the strings for a bunch of balloons, and they immediately slid out of my sweaty paw and floated off into the universe, perhaps destined to return to Earth and kill a hungry raccoon.

After everyone hugged and cried, we stood there for an awkward split second. Cali was still gathering herself, so I spontaneously decided to speak to the group. I have no idea what I said, but hopefully I conveyed our gratitude for the support and friendship and didn't make too many inappropriate jokes. Then Cali got herself together enough to speak to everyone, and halfway through, she pulled off her bandana to show off her fuzzy, little gray noggin.

The kids were there too, and it was a big cryfest.

I had invited Cali's sister and mom, but they politely declined. Even though they understood it was just a "welcome home" thing, they didn't want to celebrate prematurely. They'd wait until after the results of the PET scan in a few weeks. I wondered if I should have held off too.

CHAPTER 37
OCD, the DMV, and the ER

In 1988, my lucky number was four, but four times four was sixteen, which made sixteen *super* lucky. That worked for a while, until it occurred to me that sixteen times four made sixty-four the luckiest.

That was why sixteen-year-old Gregg was stuck at the garage entrance to my childhood home in Commack, Long Island, for so long. I had already tapped the entrance mat sixty-four times with my right toes. Right foot was good, left foot bad. Toe better than heel, so the hierarchy was naturally right toe, right heel, left toe, then left heel. Now I was tapping the doorknob sixty-four times with my right index finger. Left hand bad, right hand good, all middle fingers bad for obvious reasons, right ring and pinkie fingers okay but not great, right index finger good, right thumb best. The problem was I had to be looking to the left at the doorknob so it appeared visible in the ghosted outline of the right side of my nose. But I had glanced to the right halfway through the count, which automatically called for a complete reset and do-over from the beginning.

It was late afternoon. I had already gone through an incredibly exhausting number of rituals by now, which was normal for this time of day. My morning pee had been tricky because I could only look at the right side of the toilet. If I accidentally looked into the water, at the left side of the bowl or, God forbid, into the drain, the day was screwed. My shower took forever, from choosing a lucky towel that felt right for the day to repeatedly tapping my right foot in the tub before stepping in. There were several in-shower rituals, and then it took forever to get out. The last drop of water from the dripping showerhead needed to slide down the back of my head, off the right side of my neck, and then fall perfectly into the drain. It was best if the drip didn't touch any metal on the way in and went straight into the hole. Then I had to tap my way out of the shower, which was precarious due to the slippery tub and my lack of coordination.

The right side of the mirror was best, naturally, so I had to enter my own field of vision from the right. If I screwed up, I'd close my eyes, move back outside the view of the mirror, and enter stage right. Eventually, I just moved my position one step to the right so my face was always partially outside the frame of the mirror. Better to be safe than sorry.

Getting dressed was a high level of difficulty. The socks were key. Before I chose which went on my right foot, I would close my eyes and hold each sock to my forehead. The socks would send me a vibe, telling me which went on the right foot that day. Then I would put on the rest of my clothing, being sure to carefully follow all the rules. Finally, I would put on my sneakers, which had been lined up with precision the night before and checked several times before falling asleep. They were under my bed, with the toes lined up with the edge but the right toe slightly ahead of the left. Before leaving my room—right foot first when entering or exiting any room—and turning the light off and on the proper number of times with my right hand, entering or exiting—I would be sure to realign anything disturbed so it was at a perfect right angle. A notebook on my desk with the corner pointing at me would mean disaster. And a pen or sharp object? Forget about it. I might as well get back in bed.

The day continued. At school, I hid my requirements as much as possible. Also, some of my self-imposed rules were lifted for school, like the number of taps. Other major rules were not waived, though, like entering right foot first or avoiding major cracks or tile lines. If there was a cute girl in class, I'd be sure to look at her through the right side of my nose for good measure. And I was careful to space my class notes so a negative word did not land on the last right-hand side of the page. If I miscalculated, I would erase the offending word and move it to the next line, often rewriting the entire row so it fit properly.

There were a million other requirements and thoughts and rituals and mantras. There was counting and tapping and stepping and lining things up. There were unlucky songs, people, and objects. There were ideal words with which to complete sentences, either written or spoken. There were angles to consider, specific eyes to look through and ones to close, thumbs to be visible in a particular scenario, mantras to repeat in my head, special movements. There were numbers to avoid—three was pure evil; even was better than odd. All these things would help me control the world around me and would either mean disaster and bad luck or success and good luck.

So, that day, being a few days into the institution of the new luckiest number of sixty-four, I was particularly exhausted by the time I had to enter my house. Sixty-four was very lucky, but it was knocking me for a loop. Everything was taking longer and longer. I had screwed up the tap-count, nose-look angle and had to start over, even though I wanted to get inside the house and pee. That was when I had a revolutionary and urgent thought.

Sixty-four times four was ... what? Two hundred fifty-six? Holy shit, that would change everything.

At that moment, everything came crashing down on me. I was frozen, my hand inches away from the gold patina of the garage doorknob. I imagined the sheer torture I had in store for myself in the coming days, months, years. I became short of breath, suffocating under the implications of my new magical thought.

Two hundred fifty-six would kill me. There was no way I could handle it.

I decided I had to break free of my self-imposed chains. From this moment on, I would intentionally do the opposite of anything my mind told me. I would break the cycle and prove to myself and my controlling inner demons that nothing good or bad could happen from my rituals. There was no magic, no luck, no superstition.

I grabbed the door with my left hand and awkwardly turned it, entering my house and a new phase of freedom.

I entered with my right foot, though, just to be safe.

★★★

That was why my heart broke when Ella began imposing her own magical rituals upon herself. It started with a little foot tap here and a little touch there, but then it grew more and more obvious.

On June 28, as I waited in the car for Ella to come out of the house, I noticed her touch the doorknob several times. Then she lined up a pair of sneakers that were on the stairs. She carefully strode through the garage, stepped onto the driveway with the correct foot, and then, instead of heading for the car, she veered off to step on the walkway, then the driveway again, then the grass, and back onto the driveway before getting into the car. To anyone else, it would appear she remembered something she forgot, turned around to get it, realized it wasn't there, and then continued. Over and over. It was a strange dance, but I recognized it all too well.

She finally got in the car.

I said, "It's getting bad, huh?"

She didn't want to talk about it. She was tightly wound, as we were heading for her road test. Between driving with me and a few private lessons, Ella had become a capable driver. But she was still incredibly nervous, especially about parallel parking.

We drove, mostly in silence, to the testing site in the nearby town of Carmel. I made a mental note to help Ella with her OCD somehow.

As we got closer, I tested the conversational waters and gave some driving test advice. "You're just going to go for a little drive. Just like we do all the time. Turn here. Stop there. It's easy. Remember: blinker, mirror, blind spot." My dad had taught Driver's Ed back in the day, and I always remembered that one. "Don't forget, the test starts as soon as you get in the car. So, seatbelt on. When they say start driving, put your signal on and check your mirror and blind spot before pulling away from the curb."

We arrived at the testing area. It was a side road that led to a hilly neighborhood they used for the test. We were second in line, and we only had to wait a few minutes.

The tester approached, and I got out of the car. We had preemptively switched sides, so Ella was already in the driver's seat with the seat and mirrors adjusted. The friendly gentleman got in the car after producing a wipe from his pocket and asking me to clean the door handle and armrest for him in case I left any COVID juice on there. I stepped onto the curb, and he closed the door. I took a step back, and they sat there for a long time. I later learned the car wasn't on, and Ella was trying to put it in drive when she finally realized the problem. Bad start, but they pulled away eventually. She put her signal on first though.

I stood in the already sweltering heat of the morning, watching her drive off. My nervous little Pipsqueak driving away with a complete stranger. I could barely see the top of Ella's head through the rear window as they made the first turn, disappearing into the neighborhood. Ella was the youngest of her friends by far, having a Christmas Eve birthday. She was the last to drive and would be heartbroken if she didn't pass. I would be too, not only for her, but for me. I was looking forward to ending the driving sessions, even though they had been fun.

I walked across the street, anticipating they would return from the opposite direction. I was sweating in the heat, and it seemed like a long time before they finally rounded the corner. I was thinking about how much Cali would have liked to be here for this moment when the car pulled up to the curb and the tester stepped out after saying a few words to Ella. He nodded at me as he walked away. Out of habit, I walked around to the driver's side and stood there, waiting for Ella to get out.

She rolled down the window. "Mind if I drive us home?" she asked with a big grin.

★★★

That Fourth of July weekend, Cali had to go to the ER. Her response to the chemo had grown exponentially worse each time. By this sixth cycle, Cali was hurting worse than ever. She had been sleeping a lot and feeling generally crappy. In the past, whenever she felt queasy, Cali would pop that little dissolving pill, and it would help. The pill wasn't helping anymore.

Cali was running to the bathroom more and more frequently to throw up. She was exhausted in between sessions. Eventually, she just stayed in bed with a garbage pail and towel on the floor next to her.

One morning, I was getting dressed when Cali sat up and grabbed her stomach in pain. She had been queasy all morning and had thrown up once already, but this was new. She had a sharp pain in her lower right abdomen.

Where is the spleen? I wondered, trying to remember something I never knew.

I did know from personal experience, though, that the right side was where the appendix was. I could not imagine what a shit show it would be if Cali had to have her appendix removed right now. After an hour of hoping it was just gas and the pain would go away, I called the doctor. I got the answering service since it was the weekend.

Doctor Archie Andrews was on vacation, so the other doctor in his practice returned the call. Since the treatment center was closed, she suggested we go to the ER if things didn't change.

Things didn't change, so at 10 a.m., I drove Cali down to the hospital. We parked, walked in, and got checked into the emergency room. Naturally, by the time she was in a gown and lying in a bed, Cali's abdominal pain had subsided, and she quickly fell asleep. I sat there and stared at her.

They soon woke her up to take her blood, ask a few questions, and put in an IV for hydration. Each time, Cali listened and fell back to sleep immediately. I just sat there.

A few hours passed, and they came in with the results of Cali's blood work. Everything seemed okay, but they wanted to do a CAT scan to make sure. Cali went back to sleep, snoring lightly, as we waited. At the very least, she was getting some much-needed rest and hydration.

Eventually, they came and took her for the CAT scan. Later, they wheeled her back in, and again, she went back to sleep. We waited for the results. It turned out everything was fine. No issues.

The whole time, I was texting Shari, Cali's mom, my parents, and our kids. All on separate texts but mostly just copying and pasting whatever updates I typed. Everyone working there was more amazing than the next. The whole staff was friendly, caring, and went out of their way to make sure we were comfortable.

We got home around 6 p.m.

It was a long day. Could have been worse though.

CHAPTER 38
The Dog Days of Summer

Sometime during the holiday weekend, I reached out to John R., the guy Hunter had met and bonded with those many years ago at my niece's bat mitzvah. I knew John did well, but it turned out he was president of a huge hedge fund, so he was a candidate for my homegrown scheme to help Hunter prepare for real-world experiences. I was calling it, "Operation Expose Hunter." I immediately imagined Hunter running around in an overcoat, flashing everyone, and decided I needed a better name for my plan. Either way, I spoke to John and told him the same thing I had told Simon: Hunter was generally bummed, upset about his mom, and seeking guidance for his eventual entry into the real world.

"Operation Hunter's Smooth Entry"?

Nope.

John told me the summer interns had been hired many moons ago, and they just started the program two weeks ago. He asked if he could think it over for a bit. I figured that in a few days, he would come back to me and say Hunter should meet him for a coffee in the city to talk.

Bleh. Better than nothing, I supposed.

A few days later, John called back and told me he had shoehorned Hunter into the internship program if he were interested. If not, John totally understood. It would be remote, it was only until the end of July, and there was nothing so challenging that it would be over Hunter's head. Also, due to certain guidelines, they had to pay him. Quite a bit. He told me the number.

Holy shit! Perfect!

I thanked John profusely. Then I ran upstairs and knocked on Hunter's door. He was asleep, but I woke him up because I was too excited to wait five more hours.

His reaction was what I'd expected, which bordered on "meh." But he later seemed fired up and grateful. He scheduled a call with John for the next day to sort everything out.

That same week, Alix decided not to go to Rome. She was supposed to travel abroad in the fall, but things were stacking up against her. Even though COVID seemed to be getting under control in the States, many countries were still struggling. The school had recently announced there would be no traveling outside the country for the Italy abroad programs. While there was plenty to see in Italy, traveling to other countries on the weekends was a big draw for Alix. Then there were rumors they were going to further limit travel to only Rome. Then we heard they might impose remote learning at the institution where Alix was supposed to be taking classes. We'd be paying for her to sit in an apartment in Rome and take online classes. That was *not* happening. On top of everything, she was struggling to secure an appointment for a visa at the embassy in New York City. It all had been too much of a hassle, so she decided to can the trip and go back to Tulane in the fall.

Over the Fourth of July weekend, Alix visited Blake in Chicago. She had been looking forward to the trip but also dreading it because she knew she would be saying goodbye to him for six months. Blake was scheduled to study abroad in Cape Town in the fall for some insane reason. Well, Alix was there for an hour when she texted us excitedly that Blake had decided not to travel as well. I felt bad for them both but happy they wouldn't have to be apart for long.

Around this time, the girls decided they would go back to camp for the second session. They had seen Cali go through her final treatment and felt it would be okay. Alix would teach waterskiing as a counselor, and Ella would be a CIT (counselor in training).

I'd be sad for them to leave, but I knew it was the best thing for them. Camp is another world. Time passes differently, things are simpler, and taking care of little kids is an important experience for a young adult.

Things were really coming together for the Goldman clan:

Cali had finished her treatment.

Ella had passed her road test and was partying each night like a rabid rock star. She was excited for summer camp and then her senior year of high school.

Alix was interning and feeling good mentally and physically after a great visit to Chicago. She was also excited about camp and finally had clarity on her relationship and where she would be in the fall.

Hunter would be making bucks at a cushy remote internship and have a free month before a face-melting senior year at OSU.

Even Keanu and Loki were great. They were fed three times a day, I scooped their poop regularly, and they found a cool new string to bat around.

Then there was me.

I took a little self-inventory, considering everyone else's recent positive progress.

I was somehow getting larger around the waist and neck, despite my loose attempts at exercise, which meant I was going to have to really make an effort if I wanted to get healthy.

I was doing fine at work but was starting to feel a little disconnected from my customers. I was getting the job done, and my numbers were fine, but I just wasn't making the personal connections that came with face-to-face visits. I felt somewhat out of the loop, if there even was a loop anymore. Also, I had one incredibly difficult and miserable client who I only worked with once a year on a seasonal project, and she had been haunting me and my nightmares in recent weeks.

I was worried I was going to bankrupt our family with this pool situation on top of all the college bills and our generally large monthly nut.

I was on edge about Cali and anticipating the impending PET scan. I was also down about all the angst my kids were experiencing.

All my "New Gregg" bullshit had worn off, and I was regressing as I retreated into my shell. It had also occurred to me that certain people who reached out at the beginning of all this hadn't exactly kept up. I then began to think of others who hadn't reached out at all. The more I thought about it, the angrier I got, although I tried to push those thoughts out. I didn't want to keep score. Everyone deals with these things differently.

On top of everything, I could no longer go on social media. Our local Somers Parents Facebook group had become a political snipe-fest, and reading it raised my blood pressure to dangerous levels. Elsewhere, everyone was posting photos from their amazing lives. I would scroll through, wincing at photo after photo of people partying with their beautiful friends, drinking and laughing on boats, attending incredible events and concerts, viewing spectacular sunrises, hiking, viewing even more spectacular sunsets, and, most of all, going on vacations.

Yes, vacations. Normally, during this time of year, we'd be having a good old time. Cali and I would look forward to visiting day at our kids' summer camp in mid-July, where we would rent cabins on the Delaware River near the camp with several other couples. We would drink, Sean and I would fly-fish, and then we would drink some more, grill some food, get high around the campfire, and have a generally amazing weekend.

Oh, and we'd visit the kids at camp. Cali would always remind me about that part.

Then sometime later in the month, Cali and I would go to Maine. Or Cape Cod. Or Newport, Rhode Island. Anywhere. But *somewhere*. We'd have a chill week of hanging out poolside, eating at nice restaurants, walking around town, and maybe having some "sexy time." I'd fish, drink beer, and sleep. I'd turn off the phone. Well, I wouldn't turn it off, but I'd try to stay away from it. Cali and I would reconnect. I would feel rejuvenated. It was perfect.

That shit was not happening this summer, and it was becoming a problem. I also missed "sexy time." It had been more than a while.

Cali went in for her blood work that Tuesday, and the doctor said they were very pleased with the results. It was the first time Cali had driven herself, and she had insisted, so I stayed home. All the numbers that were supposed to be up were up, and anything that was supposed to be down was down. Scientifically speaking, of course. It was all very promising.

However, they informed her they weren't going to do the PET scan mid-July like we'd thought. They wanted to wait three *months* from the last scan, not three *weeks* from the last treatment. That would put the scan near the end of July. This meant it would be a while longer before Cali could get vaccinated. And it would be a while longer before we could do anything together out in the world. Any hopes I had of a simple getaway dissipated.

Most importantly, it meant it would be a longer wait to find out if the treatment had worked and whether Cali was in the clear.

★★★

A few days later, I was working in my office when Ella strolled by and grabbed the car keys. The big show-off with her driver's license announced she was driving to her friend's house. I bade her *adieu*, told her to be careful and to text me when she got there, and then I dove back in to work.

I lost track of time, but I suppose it was only minutes later when I heard a loud *boom* outside. This was not uncommon since every yahoo in our neighborhood was a fireworks expert lately. It was a little strange at eleven in the morning on a Thursday though. And it was July 8. Lighting fireworks now was like having the Christmas lights up in February. I went out into the garage to investigate.

Ella was sitting in the car, which was 90 percent out of the garage. The car was at an odd angle though, and the other 10 percent of the car was butted up against the garage wall. She had cut the wheel entirely too early to avoid our Jeep, which we always park at the end of the driveway. The front right bumper was crunched against the siding of the garage door. She got out and was crying, freaking out, apologizing. I calmed her down and tried not to make a big deal about it, although I was mildly annoyed.

I had her return to the car and back out of the garage, turning the wheel in the opposite and correct direction. There was a disturbing and long crunching sound as the car detached itself from the house. I examined the fallout. There was black car paint on the crushed white garage door siding. There was white house paint on the scratched front bumper of the black car. And the headlight panel was hanging off, seemingly connected only by whatever wires were in there.

Ella was freaking, out of the car again. "OhmyGodimsosorry!"

I popped the headlight panel back into place and gave it a punch with the outside of my fist. It clicked right in with an audible *snap*. Everything else would come out with rubbing compound. And I'd been planning to replace the siding and trim around the garage anyway, as it was all banged up in other places from some shmuck who was terrible at basketball.

I calmed Ella down and got her back on the horse. She drove off, tentatively.

★★★

That weekend, looking fashionable in my socks and flip-flops, I shuffled to the end of the driveway to get the Saturday paper. It must have rained for a few minutes earlier because the plastic bags were full of water. We can send billionaires into space, but we can't solve the wet-morning-paper issue.

I stood there for a moment, staring into the woods across from my house. In those woods were deer, turkeys, squirrels, raccoons, coyotes, and various other critters. There was definitely at least one bobcat in the vicinity; I had caught it on one of my trail-cams last year. I had a sudden urge to just enter the thick brush, flip-flops be damned, and live among the flora and fauna. I would give up all technology and live off the land. Maybe I'd visit Cali and the kids on occasion.

Honestly, I think I was just missing hunting season. This always happened to me around this time of year. Bow season in Westchester County runs from October 1 to December 31, so I would spend a lot of time in the woods during those months. When I was in there, twenty or so feet up a tree, the sounds of the suburbs faded and I was in my happy place. I was in the zone, looking and listening for any sign of deer, being as still as possible, but thinking about life in a meditative way. I tended to miss that around this time of year since it had been a while since the season ended.

I turned and surveyed my kingdom. We'd finally had the house power-washed, and the white vinyl siding gleamed so brightly that it seemed to glow. The light covering of cobwebs, various dead bugs, dirt, and light mildew had been nagging me every time I walked in or out of the house, and I was glad to have that off my list, even if someone else had done it. I looked at the lawn. Pretty good, but the grass was beat up along the edges of the driveway from the snowplow in the winter months. Happened every year, even though I always lined the driveway with reflective sticks. After plowing, the sticks would be cracked or buried in a drift of snow. I noticed weeds in some of the beds. I used to pull them myself, but everything made me exhausted lately, and it was too damn hot and humid.

I walked slowly back toward the house, my socks getting slightly damp from the morning dew. The garage was still banged up. The only visible wood on our house's façade was a bay window, which was painted white but noticeably rotting, as I could see when I drew closer. Also in trouble, I noted upon closer inspection, was one of the trees in front. Some type of disease had gotten hold of the tree and was slowly killing it. And something large had dug a hole right next to and, I assumed, under the front walkway. And the video doorbell had come loose, which explained why everything was at an angle on the screen when someone came to the door. And there were cracks forming in the walkway. And in the driveway.

Sweet Jesus, I needed to get back inside. I was frazzled.

I went back inside, where I quickly remembered my list of things to do was even longer. I was determined to get something off my list, so after breakfast, I spent the morning replacing the broken sliding garbage cabinet next to the sink in the kitchen with the new one that had been delivered a month ago. It was an awkward angle and a tight space, so I was bathed in sweat and grease by the time I finished. I washed my hands and excitedly walked into my office to cross it off my list.

It wasn't on the list.

How was this not on the list? I did all that work and didn't make a dent in my list?

I wrote, *Fix garbage in kitchen.* Then I crossed it off.

Boom.

★ ★ ★

Dan and Amy's pool was finally finished, and they invited us over. Cali and I initially wavered as we always did, but then we accepted the invite. We were especially pleased to learn it was just us invited, because Cali was feeling insecure about her hair and body. She trusted our good friends but didn't need to be exposed to anyone else yet. In addition to her other battle scars from her C-sections, Cali now had four quarter-sized pockmarks across her abdomen from the hysterectomy. I understood. I was not too keen on situations requiring me to be shirtless either.

Their pool had come out great, despite the wait. Everything was done perfectly. A beautifully tiled hot tub sat atop the huge gleaming pool, a relaxing waterfall pouring from one to the other. It truly was a backyard oasis. I was mildly jealous. Cali and Amy commiserated in the house for a while and eventually came swimming. Dan and I lounged in the pool all day, getting out only to take turns grabbing beers.

For dinner, Dan cooked steaks and chicken, and we ate and drank and laughed. It was a nice evening, and it gave me hope for the pool company we'd hired. They might've been backed up, but they did nice work once they got to it.

I glanced over at Cali several times during the day, just to take inventory and consciously check in on how she was doing. She looked fantastic with her silver short hair. She looked great in her little bikini, and if she was feeling insecure, it certainly didn't show. Dan and Amy have always been a lot of fun and easy to hang with, so Cali was laughing, gossiping with Amy, joking around with Dan, and in general good spirits.

Every few minutes, though, reality would tap me on the shoulder and remind me, "You don't know if the treatment worked yet, sucker."

★★★

The next day, July 11, I woke up in pain. My fingertip was throbbing, and my nail had a big half-moon, purple bruise. I couldn't figure out for the life of me what had happened.

I got up and went down to feed the kitties. I began to pop open a can of cat food and naturally hooked the pull-tab with my bruised middle finger before I had to grab a knife from the drawer to help. That was when it dawned on me. My injury was from opening many, *many* beers the day before.

Later, Ella's new driver's license was burning a hole in her pocket, so she went out to breakfast with her friend. A few minutes after she left the house, I heard a loud *boom* and ran outside. Ella had hit the garage again. Same exact spot. She had already corrected her turn and was backing down the driveway. I just waved, shook my head, and went back inside.

★ ★ ★

I went into the city on July 13. A few years ago, some of the ladies at the company had begun the tradition of taking Mitchell to lunch for his birthday. I was always a little crabby that I wasn't ever included, but I also didn't complain.

This year, someone couldn't make it. Mitchell and I had been trying to get together for lunch in July anyway, so we merged the events, and I was joining the birthday lunch that Tuesday. Which, of course, I was dreading leading up to the date, even though I was looking forward to seeing everyone. I was just anxious about leaving my comfort zone, leaving Cali alone, and the commute, really. If you could beam me to the event and back, I'd be fine.

I took the train again. Since we were meeting on the Upper East Side, I got off at 125th Street instead of going all the way down to

Grand Central and then heading back up. I then had to walk two blocks to get to the subway that would take me down to the restaurant. It was a rough two blocks full of the stink of hot urine, weed, and food trucks. Guys were lying in the street, asking if I had any cigarettes, and generally eyeballing the chump in his Vineyard Vines button-down and jeans. It felt like COVID had set New York City back to the early eighties, and it was depressing.

Lunch was nice, but it was difficult to stay focused. Nothing seemed to matter anymore except Cali's health.

★★★

Although Hunter's internship was remote, he had to go into the city on Wednesday that week, and he was not happy about it.

The first two weeks of his internship had been spotty. There were times he'd had back-to-back meetings, and other times where nothing happened for hours. The second week, he had a little work project but took care of it easily. He sat in on some calls that were interesting, and some that were over his head or boring. And my idealistic, twenty-one-year-old son had some fundamental issues with hedge funds and wealth in general. Bottom line, he wasn't exactly jumping for joy. But he was getting out of bed every morning and doing something, and I could already see a mild change in his demeanor.

Then came his mandatory visit to the city. He was increasingly crabby as the time approached. Normally, he had to be logged in at 8 a.m. and work until 5:30 p.m., so he was dreading the 5:30 a.m. train into Manhattan. I wondered how he would have handled commuting into the city every day if it hadn't been for COVID.

Wednesday came, he got on the train, and spent the day in the office doing intern-y things. The lunch meeting with the CEO was moved to the next day, and Hunter was irritated since that was the whole reason he'd gone in. He took a train home and went to bed early. He was still crabby.

The afternoon of July 15, I got a text from John R. Only your kid ..., he wrote. He went on to say that after Hunter and the eight interns had lunch with the CEO, the CEO asked if anyone had any questions.

Hunter immediately put a finger up as the other interns studied their napkins. "You are incredibly wealthy. You've made enough money to last several lifetimes. So why do you keep doing it?"

Yowza. I could imagine the awkward silence before the answer.

The CEO told him that not everyone in his company had earned that kind of wealth yet, and he wouldn't stop until they did. It was like a family to him.

Good answer, although there were possibly a few holes in his story.

I asked John if that was a weird moment, and he assured me that, no, it had been a unique and insightful question, and it generated some good dialogue afterward. Plus, Hunter had been the only kid who had the balls to ask something, so there was that.

After work, they took the interns out to a rooftop bar, where, for some reason, there was a craps table. They all learned to play, which could have been an elaborate setup to see how the interns performed under pressure, what kinds of risks they were willing to take, and how they conducted themselves. But it was probably just a fun coincidence.

Anyway, Hunter wound up partying with John. He later hooked up with my brother-in-law Sean at a nearby restaurant where Hunter had a burger and some beers with Sean and his co-workers. He crashed at Sean's apartment in the city and took an early train home on Friday morning.

Things were different after that. Hunter's demeanor continued improving. He might have felt some confidence after making the intimidating trip into the city and winning over some of his cohorts. His mojo was coming back a bit. He was energized and participating in meetings, finishing projects, and attending his therapy sessions with enthusiasm.

One day, I opened a package with my name on it. Inside was a book titled *Atomic Habits: An Easy and Proven Way to Build Good Habits & Break Bad Ones.* That's a mouthful. After asking around, it turned out Hunter had ordered it at the suggestion of his therapist. I was impressed by just the simple act of ordering the book, regardless of whether he actually read it. He really was making progress and putting in the effort to drag himself out of the dumps.

CHAPTER 39
They Moved the Finish Line

We were all on edge, waiting for Cali's 1:40 appointment with Dr. Ronald McDonald, during which she would receive the verdict on her PET scan. It was Tuesday, July 27, 2021.

I spent the morning working diligently, as it turned out to be a busy morning and my sales coordinator, Kamini, was on vacation. In Greece. For two weeks. I, who hadn't taken a vacation since July 2020, was jealous. And antsy. Much like how I could tell when six months was approaching for a teeth cleaning, I felt the general funkiness brewing when it was time for a vacation. And I was long overdue.

But the morning was hectic, interrupted only by a visit from the plumber, who would eventually be connecting our natural gas line to the pool heater sometime in 2044. He arrived, and as we walked around to the backyard, I explained that the town wanted us to file a separate permit for the heater, which would involve the gas company. It was sure to delay the process even further since they were notoriously slow to show up for a simple appointment. In fact, we had waited six months for them to show up for our generator a few years back. When we got around to the meter, though, the plumber was happy. Because of the work we'd done with the generator, we had the new kind of meter and good pipes he could connect to without involving the bureaucracy. He worked with the people at the building department every day, and if they had any questions, they could call him directly. So that was some good news. I just didn't want to use up all our good luck for the day. I would have saved it all for Cali's appointment if I'd had the choice.

We had to leave the house around 12:50 p.m. for her appointment. I would finally be able to go in with Cali and meet everyone for the first time. For now, I continued plugging away at work. Hunter was up in his room, interning away. Cali had slept in a bit, watched *Good Morning America* and some Summer Olympics coverage in bed, and then buzzed around the house, keeping herself very busy. I had a nervous sensation in my stomach I was trying to ignore.

It was 12:40 p.m. I could no longer distract myself with work. Cali was in the kitchen, no longer able to distract herself either. She made a phone call. Hunter had just come down with his laptop so he could work and eat lunch at the table. As the clock slowly ticked by, and we were finally ready to leave, Hunter suggested a group hug. He stood, waiting for Cali to get off the phone.

I stood there, too, thinking about how terrible it would be if we got bad news today. Cali's journey had been tough, but in our heads, there had always been an end to it. Six cycles of treatment, and according to the doctor, she'd be done. I could never imagine going through this longer or not knowing the outcome. Not that we knew the outcome, but the doc had been incredibly optimistic. What if this continued? Things would surely get ugly. The physical toll on Cali would be unbearable. And the mental toll on us all would need to be paid. We wouldn't come out of this whole. I wasn't even sure we would now.

I began to well up a bit.

I don't know what macabre thoughts had been going through Hunter's head in those few seconds, but he also got choked up as we both stood there, still waiting for Cali to join the hug. She finally stood up and joined us, forming a circle in the middle of the kitchen. Or just a triangle, I suppose. We put our arms around each other.

Cali, being nearly a foot shorter than us, eventually looked up and noticed we were crying. She asked, "Are you crying? *Aw*, are you gonna cry in the doctor's office?" She said that last part in a sarcastic, mother-talking-to-a-baby kind of voice.

"Jesus, Cali," I said as I pulled away. "We are both emotional here, and you're just making fun of us." We just weren't on the same wavelength, but I told myself Cali was nervous and handling things differently.

I went ahead and pulled the car out while Cali got her things together. It was eighty-nine degrees and sunny out, a huge departure from the cold, snowy days when this journey had begun over six months ago. I waited for Cali and thought about how this could be my last drive to Northern Westchester Hospital. It wouldn't be, not by a long shot, even if Cali were totally cleared. But it was still a milestone, and I couldn't help but reflect. Cali and I spent a lot of time together, driving back and forth from the hospital and her treatment. We laughed, we cried, we fought, we stopped at UPS. I felt closer to her as a result.

And what was next?

Naturally, if Cali were not healed, I'd be there for her. But, despite the Delta variant of COVID that had reached the States and was throwing everyone a curveball, my situation was going to change eventually. I'd be going into the city a bit more, traveling down to the factory again, maybe even heading overseas. I'd certainly be taking customers out to lunch, dinner, drinks, ball games, and shows. I'd be entertaining them in general. That would be challenging. I'd have to enlist more people for help, driving back and forth and doing other things.

And the kids. The kids would have to go back to school, knowing things weren't over. Hunter and Alix away at college, always wondering. Ella trying to enjoy her senior year, knowing her mom was still sick. It would suck.

Then there was Al and Arlene. I didn't know how much more of this they could take.

Who was I forgetting?

Right ... Cali. She would be crushed. It would take everything she had to muster up the strength to continue fighting, go back to treatment, handle it physically and mentally. It would not be good.

There was something else.

Us.

Me and Cali as a couple.

We were doing this together, fighting side by side, carrying each other to the finish line, which had always been in sight: some undetermined time around early August. We'd go back to our lives, stronger as a couple, with newfound respect and appreciation for each other. We'd take a much-needed vacation once Cali got vaccinated. We had plans to go to Hunter's fraternity parent's weekend and catch an OSU football game in October. We were going to visit Alix in New Orleans, take a family trip over Christmas break. Cali would focus on getting her hips fixed. She could take up tennis again, and we could go for walks together, get in shape.

But what if some asshole moved the finish line? What if we didn't know where this marathon ended? What if we were just slogging along, dragging our increasingly tired bodies toward some unknown goal? I didn't know how well we'd handle it then.

Cali got in the car. On the way, we started to talk, and we still just weren't jiving. Something was off, and we kept misunderstanding each other, starting and stopping conversations. I was irritated but didn't know why.

One of us brought up the group hug in the kitchen, and I asked if she really had to make fun of me for crying.

She said I should get over it and stop being a baby.

This angered me. I pushed her on it. "Really? I'm crying and trying to hug you, and you make fun of me." *Stop it, Gregg.* "What if I *do* cry in the doctor's office? Is that a problem for you?" *Stop it, Gregg.* "I've been there for you this whole time, and I get made fun of. That's just great." *Stop it, Gregg!*

She'd had enough. She yelled, "Are you *serious* right now? Are you really starting with me on the way to this appointment?"

I told you, shithead. I finally listened to myself and stopped talking.

A mile went by, and I said, "I'm sorry."

Cali said, "It's fine. I'm freaking out. I'm handling this weird."

We held hands for a second and looked at each other. Okay, we were good. We kept driving.

I looked at our surroundings. "How are we only at the high school? This drive is taking forever."

★★★

It was a bit strange not dropping Cali off at the curb and heading over to the CVS parking lot, but I actually parked and walked in with her.

As we passed through the automatic doors, everyone at the front desk looked up and smiled. We stopped to have our temperature taken by a suspicious-looking robotic gun as everyone greeted Cali. "Cali!" they excitedly said in unison, like she was Norm from *Cheers*.

We got checked in, and Cali introduced me to everyone. I was just babbling "thanks for taking care of her" to everyone when a guy came out from the back.

Cali introduced us. "Gregg, this is Matt."

I thought Matt was the guy who used to cut Cali's hair.

Matt, a large handsome fellow, shook my hand and smiled. At least, I assumed he'd smiled. He was wearing a mask. I was startled by the handshake, considering the potential germ situation.

"This is the guy that does everything so fast," Cali reminded me.

Right, that Matt. Different than Haircut Matt.

This Matt liked to get everything done quickly. Not that he had any reason to rush, he was working a full shift anyway. But he liked to get the patients out of there. The first time Matt had administered diphenhydramine (Benadryl) to Cali, which had been part of her routine on one of the treatment days, he rapidly gave it to her instead of slowly depressing the plunger of the syringe. Cali said that one second she was speaking, and the next she was mumbling with her head in her chest, like a drooling drunk. Another time, Matt was flushing Cali's port with a saline drip that usually took a while. He came over and squeezed the bag to hurry things along. She liked him.

Cali asked, "So? How'd the proposal go?"

Matt frowned. I think. Mask again. He said, "I didn't do it. Things are weird. I need to make sure she'll say yes first, but that ring is collecting dust in my drawer."

Whoa, I thought. *They really did get to know each other in here.*

We left the reception desk, which was different than what I'd imagined, and walked past the waiting room. We went through the doors into the back area, which also looked nothing like what I'd thought, where Cali was greeted with equal warmth and love by everyone there. Cali introduced me around, and it seemed everyone knew her even more intimately than I did.

We finally settled into the room where we would meet the doctor. That room was also not as I'd imagined, with the large mahogany desk, personal photos, and diplomas. We were just sitting in an examination room. Cali explained this was where she always met the doctor, and she had never set foot in his office. So, I could still be right about the spelunking photos. I felt the room did not carry enough gravitas for what we were about to discuss.

We sat and waited. Cali and I later discovered we were both having the same thought each time we spoke to someone. *Do they know? Did they read the file?*

We waited some more. Cali sat quietly. I was sick to my stomach. I couldn't handle the suspense for one minute longer. I wanted to scream, cry, trash the room, run out and find the doctor. But then I imagined how Cali must be feeling, so I decided to take her mind off things. I fiddled with the various gadgets around the room and pretended I was a doctor. I did some funny shit with the tongue depressors. Cali gave me a courtesy laugh. I was about to break into the drawers and get really silly when there was a gentle knock and polite "hello" at the door. I sat down quickly, looking innocent.

In walked Dr. Hopewell. I recalled all those somewhat insulting nicknames I had conjured up based on one online photo. Well, guess what? He was Dr. Hopewell now. He'd always deserved my respect, but I was being weird and trying to make myself feel better by poking fun.

The doctor was a brick house. He looked to be around six foot three, had a barrel chest, and a big, fit body. He didn't look like Ed

Sheeran at all. He wore a blue button-down shirt and a dark-blue tie with khaki pants and a white lab coat. He had a big, kind face and a red beard. He looked like a goddamn Viking—a Vikings football player or an actual Viking, take your pick.

As he sat down, he immediately began summarizing where we were in the process. He reminded us of what had initially caused him concern: the needle biopsy, the removal, and the analysis of a lymph node. It was all leading up to what I assumed would be his big announcement that Cali was cancer-free.

He reached the early Paleolithic Era when Cali interrupted. "Do I still have cancer or not?"

He looked at her with a kind, tight-lipped smile and cocked his head to the side. "Well …"

Oy vey.

The doctor continued. He explained how and what the PET scan measured, which was less of an X-ray and more of a measurement of activity. I imagined those military drone images of Kabul where they switched from a satellite image to an infrared heat display. The satellite image would be grainy and black-and-white. You'd see some tents surrounded by sand. Maybe a vehicle or two. Switch to the infrared. The screen would turn greenish. There would be red blotches of heat moving around and showing activity. One without the other would give you limited information.

So, everything looked great *except* … there were two areas causing the doc concern on the PET scan. One was in Cali's hip area. There was a lot of activity there. Could it be cancer? Anything was possible. But he didn't think so and wanted to rule it out. Most likely, it was arthritis or something degenerative. We knew Cali had bad hips that would eventually need to be replaced, so that made sense.

The other area of concern was Cali's lower pelvis. There were very small lymph nodes there, roughly half a centimeter, that were showing mild activity. The doctor said if he pulled one hundred people off the street and performed a PET scan, fifty of them would have this activity, and it wouldn't be cause for concern. However, given Cali's situation, he wanted to keep an eye on that area. The nodes were so small that he probably couldn't take them out surgically if he wanted to, but we had to monitor.

He wanted to schedule an MRI and compare it to the areas of activity. I figured this would be like laying the military infrared video over the satellite imagery to say, "Okay, that red blob we were about to nuke is actually just a wayward camel." Or vice versa, if it turned out to be the head bad guy carrying a rocket launcher.

Cali and I both let out a long sigh at the same time. It was not a sigh of relief but rather of exasperation. This was not the celebration we'd expected, nor was it the definitive conclusion we hoped for.

"What can we, like, tell people?" I asked.

Maybe it was a silly question, but we had both daydreamed about sending out a triumphant and straightforward message to the world that Cali was cancer-free. We did not imagine explaining half-centimeter lymph nodes and some activity causing concern in the hip with things otherwise looking good but infrared camels and no real way to say for sure, and we were going to do an MRI and yada yada.

The doc said this was very good news, and that even if he had seen nothing, he wouldn't say Cali was cancer-free anyway, until after five years of monitoring.

That would have been nice to know in advance. Maybe manage our expectations a bit.

We walked out of there shell-shocked. We didn't say much to each other, even once we got in the car. We didn't want to call anyone, because we didn't really know what to say.

Imagine it were the end of the Super Bowl, and the referees just told everyone they played great but they weren't sure who won. Maybe they'd rewatch videos and decide in a few years. The fans would fucking tear the place down. That's how we felt.

CHAPTER 40
Montauk: The End

In August, just when we thought it was down, COVID started making a resurgence, like Hulk Hogan toward the end of a brutal cage match. I suspected people weren't going to conform as easily this time around. That ship had sailed, and people were going bonkers about having to put masks back on or being told they had to have a vaccine. It had the potential to get ugly, especially with the return to school looming ahead.

Earlier in the month, Cali had finally gotten the insurance approval and appointment for the MRI. Naturally, her appointment with Dr. Hopewell to get the MRI results could only be held when I had to be out in Montauk for our annual company sales retreat. Our girls were still at camp, and, to my surprise, Hunter had agreed to come out east with me. I felt bad leaving Cali alone, but her mom would join her, and that would be good for them both. It may seem like a strange move, but we were all so emotionally spent at that point, and I had missed so many work-related things, so it's just what we did. We didn't have much faith in a definitive answer anyway.

The sales retreat wasn't officially beginning until Monday evening, with the bulk of our meetings scheduled for Tuesday. We would have a final dinner Tuesday night and depart Wednesday morning. Mitchell was nice enough to extend an invitation to Hunter for dinners, and he would just chill at the resort while we were in meetings. It was all usually very casual.

We arrived at Gurney's Star Island on Sunday, August 8. On the ride out, Hunter and I conversed easily, and I made a point to not bring up any major life or future-related subjects. We checked into the hotel and almost immediately headed back out to meet a customer for dinner. Mitchell and his lady friend, Amelia, were meeting us too.

We had a great time. My customer, Joe, happens to be a very cool guy, and he engaged Hunter in conversation all night. Mitchell and Amelia were awesome, and Hunter was just being his old self. He has a natural and easy way about him, and I never worry something stupid is going to come out of his mouth. He is smart enough to be able to read the room, too, so he can adapt well without compromising his true personality.

After a great evening, we rolled back to our hotel, which was right on the water and had several long docks filled with incredible boats. We weren't tired yet, and it was such a nice night, so I suggested we take a walk.

As we walked out onto the main platform from which all the other docks ran, we passed a single table on our left where a lone young woman sat, drinking a beer. She was very attractive but seemed sad, slouched over a bit and taking swigs out of the bottle. She made quick eye contact with Hunter and looked away. Hunter and I looked at each other. We said nothing and continued walking.

The night air felt extra fresh. We walked slowly down the dock, passing under white, hanging string lights overhead. We watched the boat people living their boat lives. They dined with friends on the backs of their massive, immaculate vessels, pouring wine and laughing, light music playing, glasses tinkling.

At the end of the dock, we turned and walked back, admiring the sounds, sights, and smells. One of the outdoor bars was hopping back on land, and again, we heard the clinking of glasses and jovial sounds of people interacting as we approached the pale glow of the resort lights. We passed the sad-looking woman, this time on our right. Again, she made brief eye contact with Hunter.

Or was it me she was eyeballing? Maybe it was me! It was not me. We walked on a few more steps, and I said, "She looks lonely."

Hunter said, "And sad. I think I'll go cheer her up."

I thought he was joking, but he broke away and began walking back toward Sad Samantha. He looked back and paused. "Don't wait up."

That cocky motherfucker.

I walked down the dock fifty yards or so and sat at one of the outdoor bars that was already closed. I was not in Hunter's direct line of sight but could see him from where I sat. He was standing next to the woman's table. I checked a few work emails, figuring Hunter would strike out quickly and I'd walk back to the room with him. I got sucked into a few more emails and lost track of time. I looked at my watch and noted that a half hour had passed. I glanced up and saw Hunter was now sitting. They had two fresh beers somehow. Hunter was gesturing wildly as the woman laughed, throwing her head back and exposing her neck in the moonlight.

I went back to the room.

Hunter didn't return until 4 a.m. Mojo officially replenished.

I was happy for him. He had come a long way back to the land of the living since he returned home. I hoped it stuck.

Hunter and I slept in on Monday, went to breakfast, and walked around Main Street. It was overcast and slightly rainy, so we weren't hitting the beach or pool as planned. By noon, we were back at the resort, wondering what to do with ourselves. We were just killing time until the phone call with Cali to get the results of the MRI.

At 1 p.m., Cali called me on speakerphone with her mother and Dr. Hopewell in the room. I later learned they had already been talking for a minute when Cali remembered she had a husband who wasn't on the phone, so she made everyone pretend they hadn't started yet and called me.

Dr. Hopewell said the activity he'd seen in the hip on the PET scan when overlaid with the data from the MRI told him there was major arthritis or degeneration in that area, which we knew already.

Cali asked, "Could there be cancer in there?"

The doctor said it was possible, but there was no way of knowing without an incredibly invasive, painful, and risky method of biopsy, which he did not recommend. The chances were slim anyway, and he preferred Cali see an orthopedist who would do a CAT scan. I figured they had enough scans to build a 3D model of my wife at this point, but what the heck? Cali would make a great nightlight after all this radiation. The ortho would probably offer some pain management and physical therapy until the time was right to do a hip replacement years from now. Unless it was cancer, which they couldn't tell. I felt like a puppy, endlessly chasing its tail.

Bottom line, Cali was cleared. There would be no more treatment. The doctor wanted to see her in a month for some blood work and then wait three months until the next scans. But Cali had responded incredibly well to the treatment, and it was over ... for now.

That's the best we're going to get, I thought as I hung up the phone.

I looked at Hunter, who was sitting on his bed. He'd heard the whole thing. He exhaled a breath he might have been holding for the last ten minutes. I exhaled a breath I might have been holding for the last several months.

We hugged, crying a bit.

"She's good," I said, my words muffled into his neck.

"She's good."

EPILOGUE
Monday, September 6, 2021

It was Rosh Hashanah, the Jewish New Year. We aren't religious, but you can bet your ass we gather with Cali's family for every Jewish holiday. Rosh Hashanah, Yom Kippur, Passover. I keep expecting a gathering for Tu Bishvat, the Jewish Arbor Day.

Cali and I finally made our way from the kitchen into the dining room. You'd think they'd never seen each other the way this group could yenta it up. Cali and I wrangled everyone together, politely interrupting a conversation between Shari and her mother at the kitchen table and getting Aaron and his daughter Emma out of the living room. I helped Big Al up from the couch. His knee had been bad lately, and I could tell he was hurting, even though he'd never admit it. He winced as I gently pulled him off the couch.

Hunter had gone back to school. He was still totally energized, killing his schoolwork, and partying like Keith Richards. He was already proactively working on his job search for next fall, and I couldn't have been more pleased that my little buddy was happy again.

Alix was back home with us. I had flown down to Tulane with her before school started and helped her move in; meaning I put her bed, desk, and dresser together in between eating and drinking anything and everything in New Orleans. Two weeks later, Hurricane Ida blasted the Gulf Coast. After scrambling to find flights home, Alix declared she would instead be driving with a group of friends to stay at some dude's monstrous house in Atlanta. So, she partied in Atlanta for a few days, sending us rosé selfies from the back of a giant inflatable swan in a massive pool. Then they drove to Miami and did it all over again but on someone's huge boat. Tough life. She eventually got partied out and flew home. She would stay with us until things got cleaned up in New Orleans, the power was back on, and it was safe to return.

Ella was still fired up from our college visits during the last week in August. The two of us flew down to North Carolina and hit four schools as we drove west to Nashville. It was great for her to see the campuses in person as opposed to the virtual tours we had *not* been doing. She was loving her new job at Bobo's, a local café, and the senior-year parties and events were in full swing.

Cali was great. She had put on a few much-needed pounds, and it suited her. Her skin had a healthy glow from the sun and from … well, being healthy. Her hair was a stunning pepper of light silver and dark gray. It had grown about an inch long and looked very hip. Her green eyes popped more than ever against the color of her hair. I wanted her to keep it that way; it looked so cool. Although she said she didn't, she must have liked it a little. She started that evening wearing her wig for the first time and took it off after an hour. Most importantly, that constant hint of worry was no longer furrowing Cali's brow. Sadly, it was replaced with an occasional wince of pain as she walked or a grimace when she stood up. Her hip had no cartilage left, and it was incredibly painful. And she had terrible arthritis, especially in her hands. She would be starting physical therapy the next day and was getting a cortisone shot in a week, so hopefully that would provide relief. She would need a hip replacement, but Dr. Hopewell didn't want her to have surgery anytime soon.

I was there too. My customers had moved their return-to-office date to February, so I wasn't going back to the city yet, which was both good and bad. I missed the social aspect of my job. Health-wise, I had blown off that last heart scan, and they stopped calling me to set up an appointment after a few tries. I hadn't made any significant or lasting changes to my diet or exercise routine. In fact, after Hurricane Gregg had torn through New Orleans, North Carolina, and Tennessee in late August, it would take a while to recover.

New Gregg was also a faint memory. I was back in my cocoon. If we must continue using the tired metaphor, maybe I had sprouted a pair of wings, but I was no butterfly. I was a moth, maybe. Either way, it was a slight improvement. I did have a heightened appreciation for most people.

When we finally got everyone settled in the dining room, it was still impossible to get anyone's attention. Tradition dictated that Big Al say the prayer over the bread, which was a giant challah I couldn't wait to tear into. He stood there, knife in hand, his face turning a little red as everyone yapped on and on.

"Yo!" Big Al bellowed, loud enough to startle a large gymnasium full of high schoolers.

We all quieted down.

He began. "*Baruch atah, Adonai Eloheinu melech haolam, hamotzi lechem min haaretz,*" he mumbled quickly and somewhat angrily. Maybe he hated bread.

"Amen," we all said obediently.

Before anyone could start yapping again, I raised my glass and said, "Happy New Year, everyone! Thanks for coming."

There were pleasant mumbles of acknowledgment in return.

Turning toward Cali, I continued, my glass still raised. I hadn't planned this but felt it was time to make an official proclamation about the end of Cali's long journey. "Cali, I cannot imagine what you went through this past year. But you handled it with incredible strength, bravery, and grace. I'd be a total disaster if it were me."

Everyone gave a courtesy laugh. I'm so amusing.

"Anyway ..." I stumbled.

How do you sum up what Cali just survived? How do I say how proud I am to have been by her side? I guess you just say it.

Choking back tears, I simply said, "I can't even begin to describe how proud I am to have been by your side through it all. You are simply amazing."

I'm not sure how much of that was intelligible.

Everyone was a little quieter as they clinked glasses.

★★★

Later, my ADD was kicking in, along with the five glasses of wine I had crushed. The meal was wrapping up, but the fervent conversation continued. As usual, I was all talked out and tired of trying to get a word in. I sat back, full of matzoh ball soup, challah, turkey, brisket, stuffed cabbage, meatballs, cranberry sauce, and noodle kugel. And wine. I pushed my plate away, noticing I hadn't eaten the string beans.

I sat back, observing the family. Talking, interrupting each other, gesturing wildly. Big Al sat stoically, just watching and listening. The kids were at the end of the table on their phones, occasionally showing each other a funny Snapface or whatever. At one point, Hunter video-chatted Cali from Ohio and said hello to everyone. I had texted him earlier and told him to, as he was unaware it was even a holiday, but still, it was nice.

I looked over at Cali the Silver Fox. She was in her element. Laughing, sharing stories, surrounded by family. And healthy, mostly. Exactly where she wanted to be.

I looked beyond Cali, out the front window. There was a light breeze causing the branches to sway. It had been cooling off the last few evenings and would hopefully continue.

I was looking forward to it.

I loved this time of year.

AFTERWORD
Wednesday, March 1, 2023

In February of 2022, Cali got sick again. We were so shell-shocked and horrified when we got the news, it didn't even occur to me to write about it. I couldn't find the humor in anything, couldn't see a light at the end of the tunnel, and could barely find the strength to push on. Cali was devastated. So were the kids, our families, and our friends.

The science has been evolving so quickly, though, that even as Cali completed treatment the first time around, new options had become available, including a stem-cell transplant. Our insurance company required us to change hospitals for the new treatment. Our new doctor at Mt. Sinai in New York City was just as incredible as Dr. Hopewell, and they worked together in conjunction. After several rounds of chemo, Cali had her stem cells removed during multiple procedures. She then had a multiweek stay in the hospital where she endured even more intense chemo followed by a stem-cell transplant. They actually refer to the day of transplant as "Day Zero" and count up from there because her immune system was essentially reset to that of a newborn infant.

Somehow, we all found the strength to support her. Mostly because of the example Cali set for the rest of us. After the initial shock wore off, Cali rallied herself and her troops for another fight. She dove in and fought through things I cannot even fathom.

In April 2022, Cali finished her treatment. Three months later, her follow-up PET scan was clean. And three months after that, her scan was clean once again. As I write this, we are at day 322 since her stem-cell transplant. Cali has gradually been getting all her immunizations from infancy again. While our new doctor has reiterated the five-year rule for officially being able to say Cali is "cancer free," he did say we can really celebrate after year two, April 2024. Statistically speaking, she's not as likely to relapse after that. Plus, there are now even newer treatments, like Car-T Cell Therapy, which essentially teaches your own blood to fight the disease through genetic modification; just incredible.

Self-pity isn't her thing, but one night when Cali was feeling particularly down, she cried to me, "Why me? Why me?" And while I am not a religious man, I gave her a standard line, "God gives us what we can handle." I never believed that, although it fit for Cali. Plenty of people who can't "handle it" get cancer. Cancer, while preventable or avoidable in some cases, is generally just a completely horrible, random thing. The odds of getting non-Hodgkin lymphoma are one in forty-three for a man and one in fifty-three for a woman. If you had a stadium full of fifty thousand people, you could fill an entire section with people who were going to get it.

Although Cali—and the rest of us—went through hell, we consider ourselves lucky. She survived. *We* survived. Cancer not only kills, it breaks up families and causes lasting psychological trauma. To come through it is no small feat.

On the flip side, cancer can bring people closer together. It can teach us what's really important in life and what we're truly capable of; I know that was the case for us.

Cancer is also weird. People don't like to talk about it, don't always admit when they have it. I personally didn't have many close resources to go to for experience or guidance. If this story helps just one person power through a cancer diagnosis or gives strength to a caregiver or family member, it will have been well worth the effort.

ACKNOWLEDGMENTS

For a guy who thought he lived in a tiny bubble, I was overwhelmed by the support we received. Here's thanks to anyone who reached out, sent their love, and, most importantly, sent food.

Thanks to everyone at Arkay Packaging who supported us during this time: Mitchell Kaneff, Walter Shiels, Brian Hopkins, Kris Koertge, Kamini Advani, Ruth Rugoff, Frank Clark, Jerry Duckett, Freddy Vega, Charlie Zilavy, Stephen Viola, and many others. In all fairness, I hadn't really broadcasted what was going on, so half the people I work with didn't even know what was happening.

The same applies to my customers and industry friends, but thanks to any who knew and sent their support: Nicole Flickinger, Laura Armani, Debbie Silverman, Tammy Shaw, Cindy Graney, Heather Clark, Quinn Trinh, Sara Clasen, Kim O'Brien, Arthur DeGrandpre, Gordon Ellis, Erin Teeple, Alex Boulay, Brandon Chang, Laurent Frayssinet, Joe Licari, Rob DiPalma, Kelsey Johnson, Maggie McLean, Michael Weinstein, Bob Adago, Georgianne Baran, Kerrie Griffin, Brian Bridges, Jesse Chertoff, Derek Bonham, Stu Schrode, and many, many more.

To my buddies who came out of the woodwork—Robert Gerstenfeld, Bruce Bernstein, Adam Gollance, Michael Jackowitz, Michael and David Strauss, Mike and Jon Biren, Justin Weiss, and many others—thank you.

My sincere gratitude to the group of friends who love Cali and tolerate me: Brenda and Michael Yates, Amy and Dan Ellison, Jenn and Paul Kisslinger, Jody and Darrin Klayman, Livia and Simon Pearce, Amy Kass and family, Tracy and Glenn Hechler, Jessica and Lee Goldberg, Stacey and Jason Piken, Tracey and Michael Riger, Amy Harwood, Lauren Kittridge, Laura Parisi, Dina and Chris Fabry, Alison and Bill Pepe, Maddie and Bryan Hackmeyer, Caren and Bernie Vogel, Wendy and John McCullough, Heather Monachelli and family, Carol Kalajian, Lucy and Ash Korham, Paula Chamoun, Adrienne and David Vogel, Kristin Wagner and family, Gwen Rothschild and family, Michelle and Mike Kovalyk, Stephanie Schoffman and family, Karyn and Lon Gitler and family, and Deena and Bruce Cohen. Also, Cindy Musoff, Merrill Mager, and Cali's childhood camp friends.

Thanks also to all the family members who lent their support: Harriet and Frank Finkleman, Linda and Dennis Robi, Nevin Robi, Phil and Merril Krell, Elliott and Fran Levine, Dianne and Richard Berger and family, Joyce and Corey Aronin and family, Barbara and Mitchell Dworkin, James and Ilene Nolish, and many others.

Sincere thanks to the incredible team at Warren Publishing, who massaged this lump of clay into ... well, a nicer lump of clay. Seriously, your feedback and support were invaluable. Thank you, Melissa Long, Amy Ashby, Erika Nein, Mindy Kuhn, and the entire crew.

My everlasting gratitude goes out to the wonderful people at Northern Westchester Medical. You made Cali feel safe and cared for as you gave her the best care. And Dr. "Hopewell," thank you, sir. And sorry. You are just amazing.

Most importantly, thanks to our immediate family: Allen and Arlene Leibowitz, Allan and Arlene Goldman, Shari and Aaron Fruhling and family, Bryan and Imma Goldman and family, and Sean and Lisa Leibowitz and family—not too Jewish sounding of a crew.

Special thanks to my core: Hunter, Alix, and Ella for your strength and support. We're sorry you had to go through this.

Thanks to the cats, Keanu and Loki, for being completely oblivious but bringing us smiles.

And of course, thanks to Cali, who supported me as much as I hope I supported her. I thought Nana Ruth was tough. You take the cake, lady.

If I left you off this list, it's my fault, not yours. My memory ain't what it used to be.

Printed in the USA
CPSIA information can be obtained
at www.ICGtesting.com
LVHW091129100524
779689LV00001B/90